THE *SAFE* *USE OF* HERBS

How To Use Common Household Herbs To Help You Stay Well

By **Beverly E. Coleman**, MPH, L.Ac.
Nutritionist, Acupuncturist and Herbalist

Illustrated By Gonzalo Duran

A 𝕟𝔸𝘾ℍ𝔼𝕊 PUBLICATION Sedona, Arizona

A NOTE TO THE READER

The information contained in this book is for educational purposes only. Neither this nor any other related book should be used as a substitute for qualified diagnosis, care and treatment. In the event of illness (See *The Wellness Checklist* on page xii), consult a medical practitioner (*See Appendix*). Any applications of the procedures or suggestions set forth in this book are at the reader's discretion.

First Edition
ISBN 0-9639722-2-7

Library of Congress Catalog Card Number: 93-87275

Publisher's Cataloging in Publication
(Prepared by Quality Books, Inc.)

Coleman, Beverly E.
    The safe use of herbs : how to use common household herbs to
help you stay well / by Beverly E. Coleman; illustrated by Gonzalo
Duran. -- lst ed.
    p. cm.
    Includes bibliographic references and index.
    Preassigned LCCN: 93-87275.
    ISBN 0-9639722-2-7

    1. Herbs--Therapeutic use. 2. Pharmacognosy. 3. Health
promotion. I. Title.

RM666.H33C65 1995   615'.321
                          QBI94-21173

 A **NACHES** PUBLICATION Sedona, Arizona, 1997

Cover design by Reem Hammad
Book design by Gayle R. Brodie

Printed in U.S.A.
9 8 7 6 5 4 3 2 1

ACKNOWLEDGEMENTS

For the information and ideas on these pages, my deep appreciation goes to all of my life's teachers including my Family, Friends, Instructors, Patients and the various cultures in which I have lived.

For their invaluable assistance in producing this book, special gratitude goes to the artists, Gayle R. Brodie, Gonzalo Duran and Reem Hammad, who worked tirelessly; to my mother, Delores Coleman, and to the following people: Marie Branch, Oscar Brashear, Crystal Bujol, Dorothy Jean Collins, Margot Dashiell, Rehema Gray, Alfred Ligon, Marge Nichols, Aldolfo Soto, Michele Vela, Renee Rolle-Whatley and Ora Williams.

CONTENTS

FOREWORD... vii

BEFORE YOU BEGIN THIS BOOK... ix
How It Differs From Other Herb Books.. xi
Ideal Wellness Checklist xii
Prevention and Wellness xv

ONE: **THE SAFE USE OF HERBS** 1
How Herbalists Use Medicinal Herbs Safely............................... 2
How You Can Use Common Household Herbs Safely 4

TWO: **A NEW WAY OF LOOKING AT THE BODY**..................... 7
Every Body Is Different - To Strengthen Physical Weaknesses....... 9

THREE: **INTERNAL IMBALANCES**... 13
About Internal Imbalances.. 14
Internal Heat, Coldness, Dampness, Dryness 16
Imbalances From Self-Abuse and/or Neglect............................. 24

FOUR: **EXTERNAL INFLUENCES ON INTERNAL BALANCES** 27
About External Influences... 28
Herbs/Foods Containing Toxic Chemicals 29
Cold and Hot Winds 30

FIVE: **THE ELIMINATION OF WASTES AND TOXINS** 35
Internally Formed Body Wastes 36
Internal Detoxification Of Pollutants... 38
How Wastes Are Eliminated From The Body............................... 40
The Disease and Elimination Crises 42

SIX: **HOW TO ENCOURAGE THE BODY TO ELIMINATE WASTES** 45
Via The Skin, Lungs, Kidneys, Liver and Bowels........................ 46

SEVEN: **DICTIONARY OF COMMON HOUSEHOLD HERBS** 57

EIGHT: **SCIENCE OF PREPARING COMMON HOUSEHOLD HERBS** 95
Rules For Using Household Herbs 96
How To Prepare Herbs 98
Use Herbs In Purposeful Combinations 100

NINE: **THE ART AND SCIENCE OF PREPARING MEALS
WITH COMMON HOUSEHOLD HERBS**..................................... 103
Meal Building Guidelines For Wellness 106

TEN: **RECIPES FOR WELLNESS** 109
Beverages, Grains, Vegetables, Soups, Spreads, Salads
and Salad Dressings, Sauces, Beans, Sweets, Your Recipes 110

ELEVEN: **APPENDIX** 141
A - Multi-Cultural, Holistic Health Practitioners 142
B - Suggested Reading and Resources.. 144
C - Botanical Names For *Common Household Herbs*.................. 146

INDEX 148

ABOUT THE AUTHOR 150

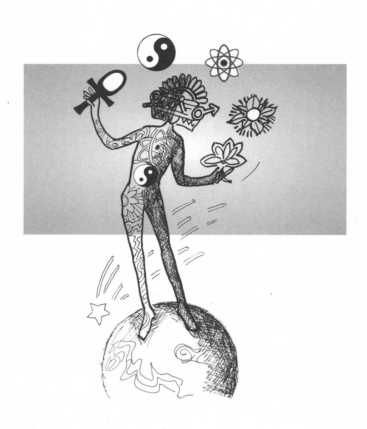

FOREWORD

There is a deep appeal in the story Beverly Coleman tells of discovering her life's vocation while living in East Africa. In the early 60's, with a degree in sociology/anthropology, she joined the Peace Corps where she was assigned to a remote village in Tanzania. There, she was informally adopted by a local family. The patriarch of this family, respectfully called Mzee ("Old Wise One"), was a school teacher during the day. By night he was a traditional doctor who set out to treat the many sick people who came from far and near to draw upon his herbal prescriptions, small bundles of herbs carried about in a wooden chest.

In her observations of the usefulness of herbs, Beverly noted there was almost no high blood pressure, diabetes, colon cancer, heart attacks or many of the other chronic diseases that plague people in the United States. By example, African villagers taught her how entwined the frame of mind and style of living are with the body's state of health.

By the time I met Beverly in the late 60's, she had returned from the Peace Corps and was beginning the formal study of conventional health care within the United States. With a fellowship for graduate studies in public health, she pursued research in nutrition, the aging process and behavior sciences. After obtaining a Master's in Public Health, she focused her studies on alternative health care philosophies and therapies including herbology, therapeutic massage and acupunture.

No matter how challenging the route, for 25 years she has been guided by her quest to gain inclusion for holistic healing approaches usually overlooked by the bio-medical establishment.

Thus, it is a sheer pleasure to see the fruits of her life's journey revealed in this lovely volume. Not your ordinary garden variety how-to guide, *The Safe Use of Herbs* forms a carefully assembled mosaic of wellness promotion advisories set in a frame of cultural diversity. Like Mzee, with his wooden chest, *The Safe Use of Herbs* is a treasure whose contents present the gems she has gathered from African, Asian, early European, Native American and today's scientific cultures. I trust the reader will cherish them as much as I do.

Margot Dashiell, *Berkeley, California*

BEFORE YOU
BEGIN THIS BOOK

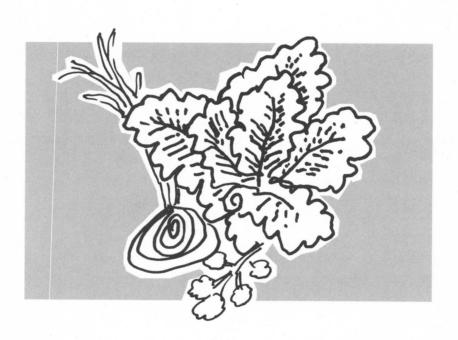

HOW IT DIFFERS FROM OTHER HERB BOOKS

The Safe Use of Herbs presents a new, enlightened, multi-cultural context for understanding the human body and how herbs can be utilized to enhance wellness and prevent illness.

Its uniqueness begins with an *Ideal Wellness Checklist* to provide the reader with the opportunity to evaluate his/her present level of wellness. In the event the results of this test indicate existing health problems, suggestions are provided (*See Appendix A*) for selecting an appropriate health care practitioner.

Even though this book illustrates how family, environment and lifestyle influence the body's internal balance, it is first and foremost a book about herbs. Its goal is to teach people how to use herbs safely.

Most herb books describe the functions and uses of herbs only from a Western point of view. *The Safe Use of Herbs* incorporates ideas and research findings from several non-Western cultures so that the reader gets a broader view of the functions and uses of herbs that are commonly found in most households.

Whereas most herb books limit the definition of herbs to medicinal roots, seeds, barks and leaves, *The Safe Use of Herbs* goes a step further. It expands the definition of herbs to include grains, vegetables, fruits, cactus and mushrooms; it considers all plant foods herbs. The *Common Household Herbs* described in this book contain specific properties that help promote wellness and prevent disease.

The Safe Use of Herbs also differs from most other herb books in that it contains recipes and ideas for enhancing the taste and wellness value of foods by using *Common Household Herbs* in a more knowledgeable and creative manner.

IDEAL WELLNESS CHECKLIST

Each question is actually a statement that defines an ideal state of health. Place a check (✓) by the statements that describe you. The responses you check will shed light on your present level of wellness. At the end of the test is a key and explanation to help you interpret your results.

1. _____ **ENERGY:** My energy level is adequate to carry out moderate daily work, exercise and personal duties.

2. _____ **REST:** I usually sleep 6 to 8 hours without waking.

3. _____ **REST:** If I am tired, I take a 15 to 60 minute refreshing rest break.

4. _____ **APPETITE:** My appetite is easily satisfied; I do not have distracting cravings or binges.

5. _____ **THIRST:** My thirst is easily satisfied by 4 to 8 glasses of room temperature fluids daily.

6. _____ **DIGESTION:** I am free of chronic belching, hiccoughs, gas and abdominal "rumbling."

7. _____ **BOWELS:** I usually have at least one bowel movement daily.

8. _____ **BOWELS:** ☎ My bowel movements are usually well formed and do not contain mucous, blood or pieces of undigested food.

9. _____ **URINATION:** I usually urinate from 3 to 6 times during my waking hours.

10. _____ **URINATION:** ☎ My urine is usually a clear/light yellow liquid.

11. _____ **URINATION:** ☎ My urine stream is forceful and uninterrupted.

12. _____ *URINATION:* ☎ My urination is free from burning sensations or other discomfort.

13. _____ *URINATION:* I usually sleep through the night without having to urinate.

14. _____ *PERSPIRATION:* I sweat only upon exertion or in warm or hot environments.

15. _____ *PAIN:* ☎ I am free of frequent or ongoing pain and/or numbness anywhere in my body.

16. _____ *PAIN:* ☎ I am free of rapid or irregular heartbeats or discomfort in the chest area.

17. _____ *DISCHARGES:* ☎ I have no abnormal discharges of mucous or blood from any of my body's openings.

18. _____ *IMMUNE SYSTEM:* ☎ I am free from chronic (frequently occurring) colds, flu and infections.

19. _____ *RESPIRATION:* I breathe easily without chest and/or sinus congestion.

20. _____ *RESPIRATION:* ☎ I do not experience shortness of breath unless I have exerted myself in some way.

21. _____ *LIBIDO:* When I am in a sexual relationship, my sexual appetite and energy are adequate to meet reasonable (one to three times weekly) demands.

22. _____ **(Men)** *SEXUAL FUNCTION:* ☎ I am able to sustain a normal erection for as long as I desire throughout sexual intercourse. And I have the ability to injaculate/ejaculate at will (rather than prematurely — or not at all).

23. _____ **(Women)** *MENSTRUAL CYCLE:* ☎ My cycle is regular; coming every 27 to 30 days.

24. _____ **(Women)** *MENSTRUAL CYCLE:* ☎ My "period" is relatively free from pain or excessive blood loss.

25. _____ **(Women)** *MENSTRUAL CYCLE:* Before my "periods" I am free of pain, recurring fevers, bloating, breast soreness or wide mood swings (PMS).

26. _____ **(Menopausal Women)** *MENSTRUAL CYCLE:* My cycle is waning. I may or may not have a "period" each month. My flow is decreasing but I am free of discomfort and excessive "spotting" between "periods."

27. _____ **(Menopausal Women)** *MENSTRUAL CYCLE:* ☎ I do not suffer from hot flashes, unusual depressions, anxieties, palpitations or chest pains.

28. _____ *EMOTIONAL HEALTH:* I avoid being overcome by anger, worry, depression, or immobilizing fear when confronted with ordinary everyday events.

29. _____ *MENTAL HEALTH:* ☎ I have a fierce desire to survive and achieve most of the goals I set for myself.

Results of a Physical Examination

30. _____ *BLOOD PRESSURE:* My blood pressure is between 95/60 and 140/90.

31. _____ *GROWTHS:* My physical exam indicates that I am free of any apparent cysts, lumps, nodules or tumors.

32. _____ *BLOOD and URINE LAB TESTS:* My lab report indicates that my chemistries are within normal ranges.

HOW TO INTERPRET YOUR RESULTS

✓ _____ *If you placed a checkmark next to all of these questions, your wellness is at an "optimal" high level. As you read The Safe Use Of Herbs, pick up pointers that will help you maintain your good health and prevent disease.*

_____ *If you miss a few checkmarks, don't worry. Your level of wellness will soon increase if you follow the suggestions and instructions in The Safe Use Of Herbs.*

☎ _____ *No checkmark together with a telephone notation means you should immediately call an appropriate health care practitioner for an appointment. DO NOT ATTEMPT TO DIAGNOSE AND TREAT YOURSELF WITH HERBS. Some of these symptoms may indicate life-threatening conditions. However, The Safe Use Of Herbs can be a helpful wellness resource to go along with your treatment program.*

PREVENTION AND WELLNESS

A surprise to many is that most illness is 60% preventable! That is, our lifestyles are 60% responsible for our health conditions. The other 40% of the responsibility for our ultimate state of health comes from:

1) Genetic factors such as disease traits passed on through family lines

2) Our mothers receiving poor prenatal health care

3) Our not receiving good nutrition and health care during early childhood

4) Social and environmental factors that are beyond our control

The fact that you inherit a disease trait does not mean you are destined to become ill. By following the ideas and suggestions in *The Safe Use of Herbs*, your general wellness and resistance (immune system) can be empowered to ward off most preventable illness. This is what is meant by prevention.

If you do happen to become debilitated or ill, you can utilize the information in *The Safe Use of Herbs* to increase your vitality and wellness level so that you regain your health more quickly. This is what is meant by promoting wellness.

However, it isn't necessary to have a disease trait or be ill in order to promote wellness. As you read *The Safe Use of Herbs* you will learn how to use *Common Household Herbs* to promote wellness and prevent illness whether you are sick or well.

ONE

THE SAFE
USE OF HERBS

HOW HERBALISTS USE MEDICINAL HERBS SAFELY

The study of herbal medicines (called "pharmacognosy") is a highly specialized and scientific area. Herbalists' (usually acupuncturists and naturopaths) formal studies usually include chemistry, biology, botany, anatomy, physiology, disease processes, diagnosis and the science of treating illnesses and enhancing wellness through the use of medicinal herbs (sometimes referred to as phytomedicines). They are then qualified to formulate herbal prescriptions based on the patient's overall medical history, symptoms and health status.

Every culture throughout the world has some sort of formal training program, including apprenticeships, through which herbalists can develop high levels of knowledge and skills. In addition, western cultures have a group of university trained scientists – called ethnobotanists – who research and write about the use of herbs in various cultures or ethnic groups. At this time, there are approximately 100 active ethnobotanists publishing works.

It is estimated that 80% of Europe's medical doctors utilize botanicals in treating patients. In Africa and South America, traditional doctors are being called upon to share their herbal cure "secrets" with university researchers. In Asia (especially China, Korea, India and Japan), bio-medical doctors and traditional herbalists often work cooperatively for the ultimate benefit of patients. 50% of the world's published works on herbs since 1992 are in languages other than English. Therefore, their discoveries, unfortunately, do not readily benefit English speaking people.

In the United States, the sale of botanical medicines has more than doubled in the last 10 years. More and more people are insisting on herbs as a viable replacement for (usually) more toxic pharmaceutical medicines. The problem in the United States is that there is not yet a centralized organization designated to provide adequate surveillance or research to assure public safety. The FDA has sometimes attempted to provide this public service but has lacked adequate staff and/or knowledge of herbs to carry out this function properly.

The FDA classifies most herbs as foods – substances that enhance the flavor and texture of other foods. According to FDA guidelines, herbs cannot be represented as medicinal substances until they have passed the rigors of modern western scientific testing. Further, they may be reclassified as non-food substances if they are found to cause harm. The FDA has classified the following herbs as non-foods; they should not be sold or used by the public as dietary supplements. Many of them are presently or may soon be classified as pharmaceuticals and their use restricted to licensed herbalists, medical doctors and pharmacists:

Foxglove (Digitalis), Belladona, Calamus Root (Sweet Flag), Chapparal, Comfrey, Blood Root, Damiana, Mistletoe, Pennyroyal, Poke Root, Scullcap, Sassafras Bark, Tansy, Sunflower Petals, Wormwood, Yohimbe Bark, St. Johnswort, Ephedra (Mahuang or Mormon Tea), Tonka Beans, Periwinkle, Mugwort Leaf, Mandrake Root, Broom Tops, Lily of the Valley, Golden Seal and a growing number of Chinese herbs

In December of 1994 the Office of Alternative Medicine at the National Institute of Health held its first national conference on the use of botanical (herb) medicines in the United States. (For the proceedings, see *Appendix B*) The role of government officials was to listen to how other countries and groups within this country use and deliver botanicals safely. The conference was held in response to the public's growing determination to use herbs to resolve health problems. And, because national health planners are beginning to recognize the role herbs might play in promoting public wellness and preventing disease. *The Safe Use of Herbs* can ultimately ease the burden on the health care system.

HOW <u>YOU</u> CAN USE
COMMON HOUSEHOLD HERBS SAFELY

Almost any edible substance might cause harm if consumed in unreasonable amounts. The key to determining what is safe and what is unsafe is knowledge. The pages of this book are filled with knowledge necessary for making correct decisions about safely using herbs. By using *Common Household Herbs* as suggested throughout this book, you may be certain you are using herbs safely and correctly.

As you read, you will discover that there are many different categories of herbs. Some are nutritive such as whole grains. Each grain is a seed, filled with its own vibrant life force. A bowl of rice, millet or other grains is actually a bowl of low-fat seeds. Green leafy and root vegetables, seaweeds, stalks and fruits are also nutritive herbs; that is, they are usually rich in certain vitamins and minerals. This group may be eaten safely in large quantities.

Another kind of *Common Household Herbs* is that which is nutritive while containing specific properties capable of altering usual internal body functions. Among this group are parsley, watercress, alfalfa, onions, garlic, ginger, mushrooms, nuts and oily seeds. It is safe to eat these herbs regularly but they should be eaten in smaller amounts unless the changes they bring about are desirable.

Yet another group is that used to season or flavor foods. This group is called "spices." Cloves, nutmeg, cinnamon, sage, thyme, oregano and rosemary are examples of this group. They may greatly affect internal body functions when taken even in small amounts. Therefore, they should be used sparingly. (The spice trade is better regulated for quality and toxicity than other herbs.)

Although many *Common Household Herbs* sometimes possess mildly medicinal qualities, their main functions are to enhance the taste, texture and nutritional value of other foods. By learning more about these herbs and how to use them, you can conveniently and effectively incorporate them into your everyday life to promote greater wellness and prevent disease.

The most important rule in using herbs safely in cases of illness is *do not attempt to self-diagnose and self-medicate with herbs!*

Many people mistakenly think that reading several books about herbs qualifies them to diagnose and treat themselves and others with herbs. They argue that the conventional (bio-medical) health care system frequently fails to resolve many of today's health problems. In seeking more effective, less expensive approaches to treatment, they go to healthfood stores and Chinese herb shops in search of herbal products to help resolve their health problems. This is usually not a safe solution.

When you become aware of anything irregular occurring in your body (See *Ideal Wellness Checklist*), the safe thing to do is seek the expert counsel of a qualified health practitioner (See *Appendix A*). While you are under the care and guidance of your choice of practitioners, continue to follow the ideas within *The Safe Use Of Herbs* in order to promote your own wellness.

A Special Note: There are many medicinal herb preparations on the market today that may be used to treat illnesses. However, the safe use of these products requires the assistance of a knowledgeable practitioner who is familiar with product reliability and safety. Most herb manufacturing companies have good reputations for following the same safety guidelines the government requires of pharmaceutical companies. Reliable herb manufacturing companies use unpolluted raw materials and standardized low heat processing methods, so that each batch is uniform in quality. Also, these superior companies staff highly skilled herbalists to formulate their products.

Unfortunately, all herb companies do not adhere to these high standards. Random inspection by the FDA have uncovered toxic substances in products, the use of poor quality raw materials and variations in processing. Products are sometimes mislabeled, and some of the imported herbal formulas from China have been found to be "laced" with pharmaceuticals. A properly informed herbalist usually knows which companies are reputable.

TWO

A NEW WAY OF LOOKING AT THE BODY

EVERY BODY IS DIFFERENT

No two people are alike. We are each born with different physical strengths and weaknesses. How we turn out is determined by our family genes. We can't change our genetic outcome but we can systematically strengthen our areas of inherited weakness.

When our bodies are stressed or challenged in any way, it is often our areas of weakness that are the first to show signs of dysfunction. That is, the organs and chemical functions within these areas are more likely to go off balance and begin breaking down. This is the beginning of illness.

To determine your area(s) of weakness, note the various symptoms listed under "Upper," "Middle" and "Lower" Body Weaknesses in this chapter. You can prevent being overcome by illness by strengthening your areas of weakness with the appropriate *Common Household Herbs*.

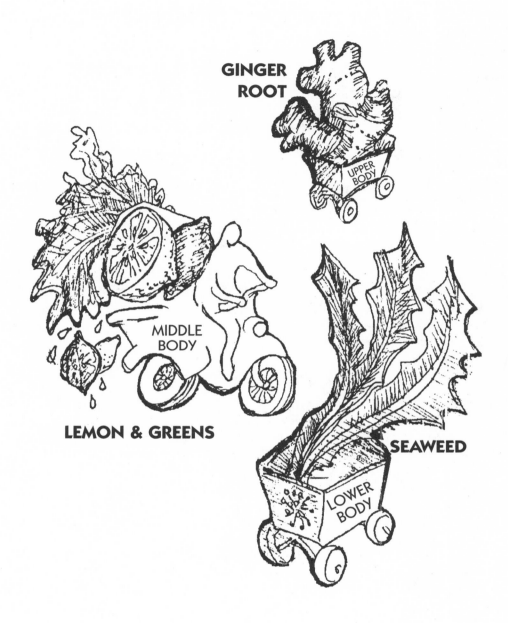

GINGER
ROOT

UPPER
BODY

MIDDLE
BODY

LEMON & GREENS

SEAWEED

LOWER
BODY

TO STRENGTHEN PHYSICAL WEAKNESSES

UPPER BODY WEAKNESS

Respiratory, Heart, Circulation, (dry) Skin problems, Sensory problems (eyes, ears, taste, touch, smell)

Strengthening Herbs

Anise, Buckwheat, Caraway, Cayenne Pepper, Cinnamon, Dill, Fennel, Fenugreek, Garlic, Fresh Ginger, Horseradish, Marjoram, Mint, Mustard Seed, Onions, Oregano, Rosemary, Sage, Sunflower Seed, Thyme, Radish (including Radish Sprouts), Watercress

MIDDLE BODY WEAKNESS

Irregular bowels, Habitual gas and/or belching, Phlegm or Mucous discharges anywhere in the body, Joint pains, Headaches, Tendency to gain weight easily, Water retention or edema, Chronic anemia, Heavy sweating and Shortness of breath even without exertion, Sensory problems (eyes, ears, taste, touch, smell)

Strengthening Herbs

Agar, Alfalfa, Allspice, Anise, Bamboo Shoots, Bay, Burdock Root, Cactus Pads, Caraway, Cardamom, Cayenne Pepper, Celery, Chives, Cinnamon, Cloves, Coriander, Cumin, Dill, Fennel, Fenugreek, Flax Seed, Garlic, Fresh and Dry Ginger, Grains, Greens, Horseradish, Mint, Mustard Seed, Nutmeg, Rosemary, Sage, Savory, Tarragon, Taro Root, Turmeric, Yucca

LOWER BODY WEAKNESS

Low back and knee pain, Frequent urination (more than 6 times during the day), Waking up to urinate at night, Swelling in the legs, Weakness in the legs and joints, Sexual inadequacies, Ringing in the ears, Normal signs of aging, Sensory problems (eyes, ears)

Strengthening Herbs

Basil, Beans (especially Black, Small White and Adzuki), Celery Seeds, Cinnamon, Cloves, Fennel, Flax Seed, Fenugreek, Dry Ginger, Grains, Greens, Marjoram, Oregano, Pumpkin Seeds, Nuts, Rosemary, Sage, Savory, Seaweeds, Sesame and Sunflower Seeds, Watercress

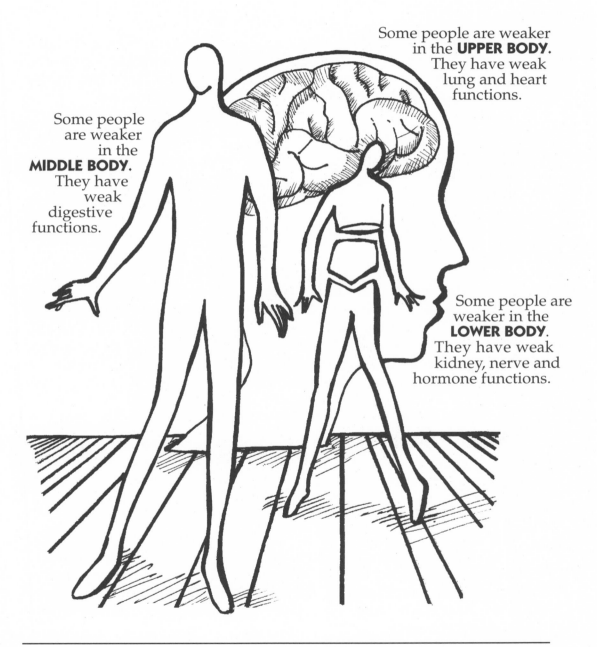

Some people are weaker in the **UPPER BODY**. They have weak lung and heart functions.

Some people are weaker in the **MIDDLE BODY**. They have weak digestive functions.

Some people are weaker in the **LOWER BODY**. They have weak kidney, nerve and hormone functions.

THREE

INTERNAL IMBALANCES

ABOUT INTERNAL IMBALANCES

As you read this section, you will be introduced to several "new" concepts about the body and the use of herbs from both Eastern and Western cultural views. Through this multi-cultural approach, you will learn how to alter internal balances and promote wellness by using *Common Household Herbs*.

First is the relationship between internal heat and cold. Many people describe themselves as "cold" or "hot" natured. These physical traits are often inborn. But most people develop these or other traits because of their lifestyles.

Another important internal balance is between water and heat. Too much dampness puts out the fire. Too much heat evaporates moisture causing dehydration or dryness. These inclinations may also be inherited or brought about by lifestyle.

Sometimes internal balance is disturbed by deficiencies. That is, the body is not being supplied with the fluids, nutrients, oxygen, exercise or rest it needs to generate energy. Or, perhaps, too much is being demanded of the body leaving it exhausted. This especially occurs when there is over-consumption of alcohol or sugar and with drug use or excesses of sexual or other physical activities. Among children such states are usually caused by prolonged illness, parental neglect or because parents do not have adequate health-related knowledge to give their children a healthy start in life.

Internal imbalances often occur in multiples. Even though you may be experiencing more than one of the imbalances in this section, one is usually a dominant or primary condition. The others are secondary. The cause of these imbalances may also be associated with "Upper," "Middle" or "Lower Body" weaknesses. That is, we are born with these weaknesses and, if our lifestyle is not appropriate to our needs, they eventually contribute to our internal imbalances.

Each internal imbalance creates its own set of symptoms. In the West, these symptoms are given disease names and treated with pharmaceuticals. In the East, however, they are considered indications of deeper disturbances. For example, excess internal dampness may be a major factor in creating lung congestion, digestive disturbances, sinusitis, diarrhea, high blood pressure, edema or congestive heart problems depending on the patient's genetic predispositions and which area of the body has become the weakest.

The body can be compared to a balance scale continuously juggling its internal environment in an effort to reach or maintain wellness. By reinstating proper internal balances, symptoms often disappear without other kinds of treatment.

There are many ways to reinstate and maintain internal balances. In Eastern medicine, practitioners use medicinal (therapeutic) herbs, many of which are highly toxic, to accomplish this task. Medicinal herbs are used after the onset of illness. Their use requires great knowledge and skill *(See Chapter One: The Safe Use of Herbs)*. In this chapter, you are introduced to an Eastern approach to promoting wellness. Instead of using medicinal herbs, however, milder *Common Household Herbs* are recommended.

Eastern medicine categorizes all herbs according to their healing and health promoting properties. For example, there are herbs that alter internal body temperature; they can be internally drying or moistening. Some herbs cause the body's energies to ascend while others have a descending effect. And, many herbs act as tonics, adding energy to a depleted body. *The Safe Use of Herbs* has classified *Common Household Herbs* in the above manner.

To reinstate or maintain your internal balance select and use the herbs that are listed on the page of your primary condition. Add one or two herbs from the herbs listed on the page(s) of your secondary condition(s). Use these herbs as suggested in *Chapters Eight, Nine, and Ten.*

SOME PEOPLE TEND TO OVERHEAT INTERNALLY

They are more uncomfortable than most people in moderately hot weather. When most people feel chilled in cool weather, "internally hot" people can go without a sweater or jacket. This condition stems from the over consumption of animal products, alcohol, fried foods, fats/oils, sweets and/or refined foods. It is aggravated by emotional frustrations. Internal pressure together with heat causes them to sweat easily. They are often agitated, irritable and impatient. They thirst for cool drinks and generally like to sleep with the windows open. The fact that heat and energy tend to rise to the head often creates headaches and elevated blood pressure.

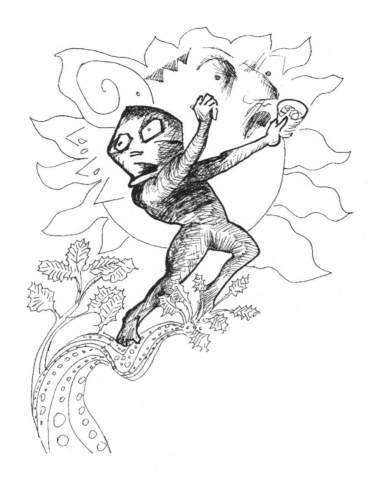

For a healthier internal balance, the "internally hot" type should limit the intake of sweets, alcohol, meats, spicy and fatty foods. Increase the intake of cooling foods:

Alfalfa, Aloe Vera, Bean Sprouts, Burdock Root, Celery, Cucumber, Grape Leaves, Greens, Lemon, Mint, Mung Beans, Turmeric, Watermelon and other Fruits, Watercress. If excess dampness (phlegm or mucous) accompanies internal heat, also use: **Bamboo Shoots, Barley, Cornsilk, Parsley, Taro Root**

OTHER PEOPLE TEND TO
BE COLD INTERNALLY

They have cold hands and feet and need sweaters or coats when it is not cool to most people. They may also have "gurgling" sounds in the abdomen and soft or loose stools. "Internally cold" people do not have much vigor or energy and they commonly complain of lower back and knee pain. They sometimes feel a heaviness and pain in the chest that is not medically diagnosed as a heart problem. And, they are often bothered by joint and muscle stiffness when the weather is cold and damp. If the pain subsides or disappears in hot weather, however, this is usually not true arthritis. It is an invasion of cold into joints and muscles that don't have enough internal heat to fight off the penetration of external cold.

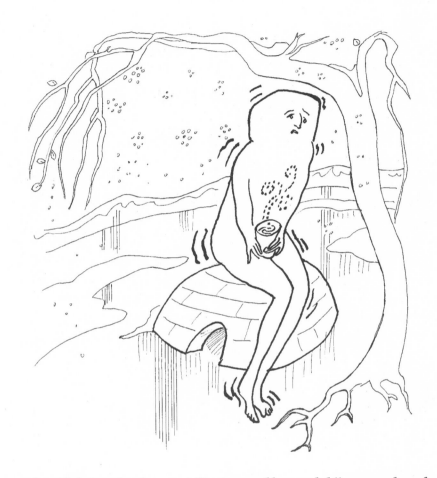

For a healthier balance "internally cold" people should limit the intake of fruits, raw and other cooling foods. They should increase the use of hot soups, cooked foods and warming herbs:

Allspice, Anise, Buckwheat, Cardamom, Cayenne Pepper, Cinnamon, Cloves, Fennel, Fenugreek, Ginger, Green Onions, Horseradish, Mustard Seeds, Nutmeg, Sage, Savory

THEN THERE ARE THOSE
WHO RETAIN WATER OR DAMPNESS

They are often bloated or puffy under the skin and tend to gain weight easily. Although they do not usually have big appetites, they crave and binge on sweets, starches and/or fatty foods. Because "water puts out fire," people who are "internally damp" or waterlogged tend to be lethargic. Their legs often feel heavy and they become sleepy at inappropriate times.

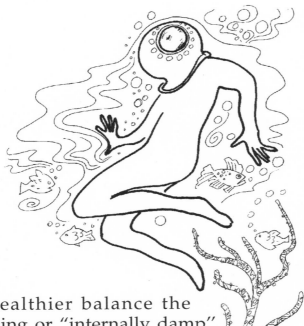

For a healthier balance the water retaining or "internally damp" type should avoid sweets and fats and limit the intake of starches. Equally important, they must exercise vigorously at least 4 times weekly. They should increase the use of herbs that help remove excess water from the body:

Bamboo Shoots, Cactus Pads, Carob, Cardamom, Fennel, Ginger, Prickly Pears, Parsley, Rice (Dry fried before boiling), **Sage, Tarragon and Watermelon Seeds.** If internal overheating accompanies a damp condition, the following herbs both cool the body and remove excess water: **Barley, Cornsilk, Parsley, Taro Root**

SOME PEOPLE BECOME
INTERNALLY DRY

This especially happens to children, older people or after a fever or long illness. "Internally dry" people are generally thirsty, constipated, have night sweats, occasional ringing in the ears and may have high blood pressure because the kidneys and liver have lost the moisture they need to work properly. Insomnia and palpitations may also occur in cases of "internal dryness."

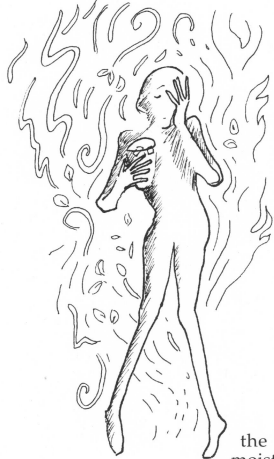

For a healthier balance,
the "internally dry" type should
moisturize and nourish the kidneys
and liver by limiting the intake of warming and spicy foods.
They should increase the intake of cooling, lubricating,
moisturizing foods:

Agar, Adzuki and Black Beans, Alfalfa, Bean Sprouts, Black Sesame Seeds, Celery, (tender, green) Coconut, Fenugreek Seeds, Mung Beans, Juicy Fruits (especially Melons, Loquats and Persimmons), Poppy Seeds, Walnuts and most Vegetables

PEOPLE ALSO
GET OUT OF BALANCE BECAUSE OF
SELF-ABUSE and/or NEGLECT

This state of physical, mental and emotional exhaustion is sometimes called "burnout." It can occur from combinations of:

- Not enough rest
- Prolonged stress and tension
- Shallow breathing
- Inadequate exercise
- Too much sexual activity
- Drinking alcohol
- Drug use
- Cigarette smoke
- Overwork
- Poor diet and eating habits

In this state, people often tend to withdraw and become disinterested in family, work and goals. It is important to seek help before illness develops. And, of course, stop doing those things that cause internal imbalances.

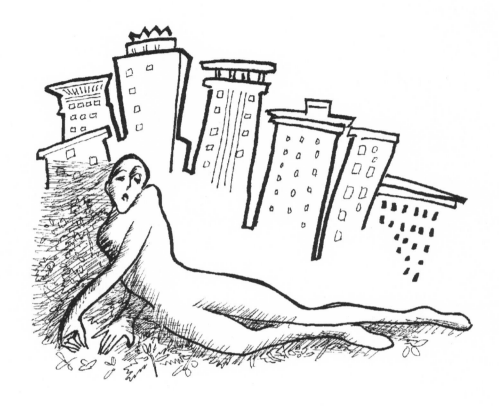

Use *Common Household Herbs* with tonic action:

Agar, Alfalfa, Basil, Celery, Cherries, Cinnamon, Cloves, (tender, green) Coconut, Coriander, Cumin, Dill, Fennel, Most Fruits and Vegetables, Grains, Greens, Lemongrass, Marjoram, Nuts (Vit E), Oregano, Parsley, Pomegranate, Rosemary, Sage, Savory, Seaweeds, Sesame and Sunflower Seeds, Thyme, Watercress

FOUR

EXTERNAL INFLUENCES ON INTERNAL BALANCES

ABOUT EXTERNAL INFLUENCES

Even though we have the power to prevent most illnesses by altering our lifestyles, there remain many external influences over which we have very little control. These external factors can also lead to internal imbalances.

Weather is one such influence. We can shield our bodies from the ravages of extreme cold and hot weather but these elements can eventually seep through cracks in our defenses — particularly if our level of wellness is not strong enough to resist the penetration of cold or hot winds. This section of *The Safe Use of Herbs* contains information about how cold and hot winds penetrate the body's defenses to cause the common cold. And, it spells out how *Common Household Herbs* can be used safely to reverse these conditions.

There are additional external factors that should be taken into consideration as they, too, can alter internal balances and wellness. These are pesticides, fungicides, preservatives and other additives used by the food industry on our food supply. They are often cancer-causing (carcinogenic). Many of them alter genes (mutagenic). Others poison or irritate the nervous system (neurotoxic).

Although these substances are outside the major focus of this book, they often determine the safety and uses of *Common Household Herbs*. Since they have a tremendous impact on our levels of wellness — causing discomforts, illness and even death — some pertinent information about toxic substances as they may affect herbs are presented on the next page. (For more information on toxic chemicals and other foods, see *Appendix B: Suggested Reading and Resources*.)

TO AVOID HERBS AND OTHER FOODS THAT CONTAIN TOXIC CHEMICALS

(Pesticides, Fungicides, Additives and Preservatives)

1. Avoid using produce grown in other countries. Most countries do not restrict the use of many toxic pesticides now outlawed in the United States. Herbs sold at health food stores and markets are often imported from other countries where they are less expensive to grow and harvest. We have no way of knowing whether or not they are sprayed with chemicals.

2. Use produce that has been grown locally at certified organic farms. These are available at healthfood stores, some specialty markets, direct-from-the-farm markets and neighborhood co-ops.

3. Do not habitually eat out. Most restaurants do not use organic produce or foods without additives or preservatives.

whenever possible...

4. Grow many of your *Common Household Herbs* either in the yard, in patio planting pots or in planting boxes 6 feet square by 1 foot deep.

5. Make your own organic fertilizer by recycling kitchen wastes into compost heaps adding leaves, grasses, earthworms, manure and water to create your own organic fertilizer. (Many chemical fertilizers are toxic.) Use companion plants such as marigolds to repel garden pests.

6. Plant berry vines and fruit trees wherever possible.

COLD WINDS CAN INTERRUPT INTERNAL BALANCES

Cold wind blowing seeks its way into the body mainly through the upper back and neck. Most people automatically protect these areas from the cold by raising collars, wearing neck scarfs and putting on hats. When the internal body is well balanced and the immune system is strong, the body can usually produce enough internal heat and energy to prevent cold wind from penetrating the skin. However, if the body is weakened by internal imbalances or the cold air attack is fierce and relentless, it cannot fend off the invasion of cold air. As cold air penetrates the skin, shivering occurs, muscles begin to resist, stiffen and ache. Headaches, sniffles and coughing usually follow. This is one of the major causes of "the common cold."

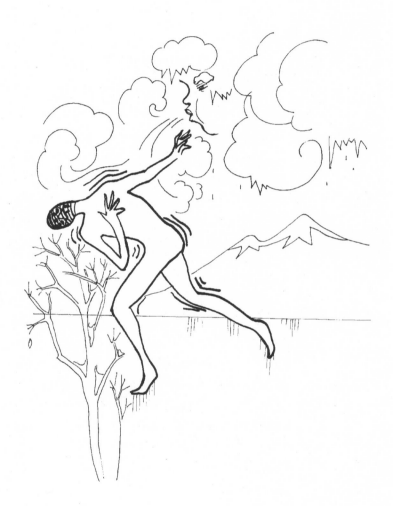

To regain internal balance from the intrusion of cold winds, immediately use:

Cinnamon, Fresh Ginger, Oregano, Marjoram, (Hot) Sage, Thyme

HOT WINDS ALSO INTERRUPT
INTERNAL BALANCES

Hot winds blow mainly in warm, dry weather. The California "Santa Anas," and other winds that blow over deserts and hot plains are examples of hot winds blowing. They dry and irritate the skin, nasal passages, throat, lungs and cause fever.

Many people "catch colds" in the summer because of breathing in hot air. This causes the throat to become dry and scratchy. The lungs rebel against dehydration by sneezing and developing a dry, hacking cough. People who are "internally dry" and who overheat internally tend to be more affected by hot blowing winds.

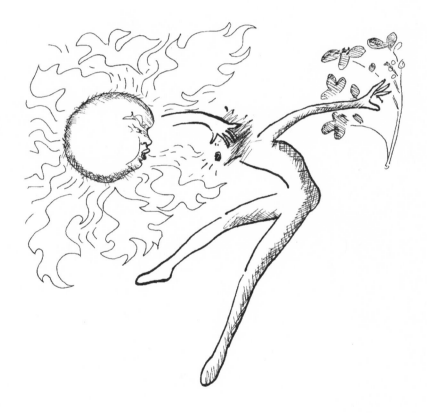

To regain internal imbalances when hot
winds bombard the body use:

Mint

FIVE

THE ELIMINATION OF WASTES AND TOXINS

INTERNALLY FORMED BODY WASTES

Before exploring how wastes are eliminated from the body, the diagram on the following page illustrates how wastes are formed when the body is out of balance. They are primarily a product of weakened and incomplete digestion. From a Western scientific point of view, internally formed wastes particularly burden the lymphatic system.

The lymphatic system is a network of vessels that run throughout the body. They contain a clear, colorless fluid in which unused particles of protein, fat and other substances are deposited and partially detoxified by "soldiers" of the immune system (called lymphocytes and monocytes). The content of lymphatic vessels is then drained into veins located mainly in the neck, chest and pelvic areas from where it may ultimately be eliminated from the body.

Because lymphatic fluid moves much more slowly than blood, it can easily become thickened (phlegm) and saturated with wastes. If the lymphatic system does not get rid of internally formed wastes efficiently for an extended period of time, they accumulate and deposit in organs, walls of blood vessels (plaque) and joints thereby obstructing the circulation of body fluids.

Accumulated waste build-ups are also perfect breeding places for disease-causing fungi, bacteria and viruses.

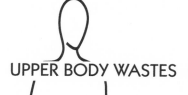

UPPER BODY WASTES

Are formed when breathing is too shallow to rid the lungs of "used" air and when the circulation of blood is obstructed or slow so that body fluids become stagnant. Poor digestion also creates phlegm/mucous wastes that rise up to burden the lungs and sinuses.

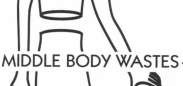

MIDDLE BODY WASTES

Are formed when digestion is incomplete thereby depriving the body of many nutrients in the food we eat. It leads to bloating and the formation of phlegm which seeks its way out of the body thru the lungs, sinus, skin, bowel, vagina, penis, kidney and bladder discharges.

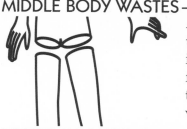

LOWER BODY WASTES

Are formed when kidney and bowel functions are sluggish – and by the downward seepage of phlegm from incomplete digestion. These wastes stagnate in the lower abdomen and pelvic area. Soft masses (called "phlegm mass tumors" in Chinese medicine) can also form in these conditions. This is *one* cause of uterine and prostate inflammations and growths.

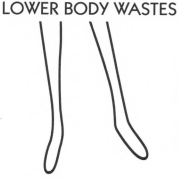

To stimulate circulation use:
> **Basil, Bay, Cayenne Pepper, Chives, Cinnamon, Ginger, Mint, Saffron/Safflower, Turmeric.**

To stimulate the immune system use:
> **Cinnamon, Garlic, Fennel, Fresh Pineapple, Broccoli/Cabbage/Carrot/Cauliflower Mix**

To eliminate phlegm use:
> **Cardamom, Ginger, Orange Peels**

For anti-fungal, antiseptic and/or anti-viral action use:
> **Basil, Cinnamon, Cloves, Cranberries, Fenugreek, Garlic, Grapefruit Seed Extract, Horseradish, Lemongrass, Onion, Fresh Pineapple, Sage, Savory, Thyme**

INTERNAL DETOXIFICATION OF POLLUTANTS

Another type of waste build-up occurs when toxic substances foreign to the body are consumed, inhaled or absorbed through the skin. Additional sources of toxins to those mentioned in *Chapter Four* are polluted air or water, alcohol, cigarette smoke, recreational or pharmaceutical drugs, chemical pollutants at the work place, many home building and maintenance supplies and materials.

The liver plays the major role in detoxifying the blood of these foreign substances. Each time a foreign substance finds its way into the blood, the liver attempts to "capture" it, break it down and neutralize it. When the blood becomes heavily saturated with foreign substances the liver is overburdened and can no longer detoxify the blood efficiently. Excess toxins are sometimes eliminated through the bowels in the fiber content of high fiber diets. They are also stored in fat cells throughout the body. Or, they travel around the body disrupting the normal balance of healthy cells.

Modern Western medicine (sometimes called biomedicine) gives very little attention to the health hazards of either internally formed waste or build-ups of toxic substances in the body. This is because the emphasis of Western medicine is on the treatment of disease rather than its prevention.

On the other hand, African, Asiatic, Native American and European "folk" medicines have traditionally been more concerned with preventing disease and promoting wellness by periodically "purging" the body of waste build-ups. This is accomplished partly by fasting or, at least, restricting the diet in various ways. (*See this Chapter: "How Wastes Are Eliminated."*) At the same time, herbs are taken that alter the quality of the blood and strengthen the liver and the body's ability to eliminate wastes. Even though these cultures came by their scientific knowledge in different ways than did Western science, they, too, recognize that the liver functions detoxify the blood.

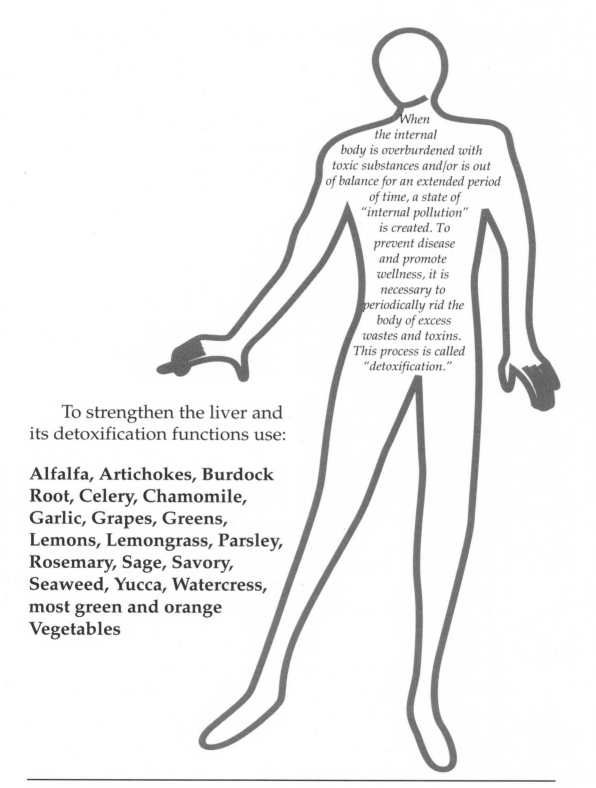

When the internal body is overburdened with toxic substances and/or is out of balance for an extended period of time, a state of "internal pollution" is created. To prevent disease and promote wellness, it is necessary to periodically rid the body of excess wastes and toxins. This process is called "detoxification."

To strengthen the liver and its detoxification functions use:

Alfalfa, Artichokes, Burdock Root, Celery, Chamomile, Garlic, Grapes, Greens, Lemons, Lemongrass, Parsley, Rosemary, Sage, Savory, Seaweed, Yucca, Watercress, most green and orange Vegetables

HOW WASTES ARE ELIMINATED FROM THE BODY

Blood flows throughout the body's network of arteries and capillaries delivering nutrients and oxygen at the "docks" of the body's cells so that they can carry out their work. The cells, in turn, give off wastes as they utilize the nutrients and burn fuel in order to create energy. Through a network of veins and capillaries, the blood then picks up these wastes and circulates to the five major "dumps" where wastes are eliminated from the body. (Veins and capillaries also receive wastes from the lymphatic system.)

When any of these elimination ("dump") sites are underactive, the normal amount of waste at that particular site is not eliminated. This places a greater burden on the remaining elimination sites. For example, if the bowels do not move regularly (at least one time daily), the skin may "break out" in an effort to eliminate more wastes. Or, the kidneys may become overwhelmed and sluggish by the extra work load.

THE 5 MAJOR ELIMINATION ORGANS IN THE BODY

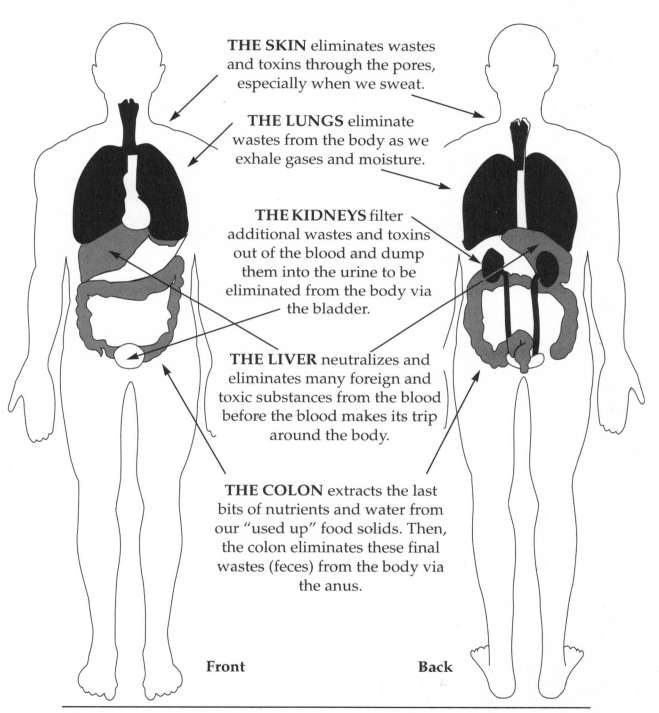

THE SKIN eliminates wastes and toxins through the pores, especially when we sweat.

THE LUNGS eliminate wastes from the body as we exhale gases and moisture.

THE KIDNEYS filter additional wastes and toxins out of the blood and dump them into the urine to be eliminated from the body via the bladder.

THE LIVER neutralizes and eliminates many foreign and toxic substances from the blood before the blood makes its trip around the body.

THE COLON extracts the last bits of nutrients and water from our "used up" food solids. Then, the colon eliminates these final wastes (feces) from the body via the anus.

Front

Back

THE DISEASE CRISIS

When the body becomes saturated with wastes and the organs of elimination are not functioning efficiently some sort of disease is certain to appear. It is impossible to constantly overload the body with toxins and internal wastes without finally reaching a "disease crisis."

In Western medicine, such disease states are given names such as arthritis, athlerosclerosis, digestive disturbances, stones, various kinds of inflammations and discharges, bronchitis, hayfever, sinusitis and frequent colds and flu. Western medicine's response to disease crises is usually treatment with more toxins — pharmaceutical medications. By so doing, diseases are rarely cured; only the symptoms are temporarily eased.

Most disease processes can usually be slowed down or reversed by making changes in the lifestyle that encourage the body to eliminate more wastes than it builds up.

THE ELIMINATION CRISIS

The "elimination crisis" appears suddenly, when a person is feeling stronger and more energetic than usual. At these times, the body has the strength necessary to "kick out" unhealthy matter. The "elimination crisis" often presents itself in the form of a three or four day cold or flu. During the fever phase, the body sweats thus releasing wastes and toxins. Muscles usually ache and there may be headaches. The bowels should be more active than usual which often leads to an increase of intestinal gases. Mucous/phlegm with foul odors may be discharged through any or all openings of the body. After the acute phase has passed, mucous/phlegm may continue to be discharged from various body openings for several days or weeks. These discharges should be encouraged because they contain wastes, toxins and, possibly, bacteria and viruses that should be eliminated from the body.

The "elimination crisis" differs from the "disease crisis" in that disease symptoms usually last longer and gradually become more intense. Disease uses up the strength and energy of a person. The "elimination crisis," on the other hand, ultimately helps a person become stronger and healthier. Many discomforts and symptoms of disease slowly disappear with each "elimination crisis." This is why some health care practitioners also call it a "healing crisis."

SIX

HOW TO ENCOURAGE THE BODY TO ELIMINATE WASTES

STIMULATE SKIN FUNCTIONS

Before bathing, use a dry natural bristle brush to vigorously brush the entire body skin surface. Dry skin brushing stimulates blood flow and skin functions. Bathe with a loofah sponge to remove dry, dead skin. Take alternating hot and cold showers to bring blood to the skin surface where it can eliminate wastes through the pores.

CAUTION: Saunas and jacuzzis serve the same purpose but **should not be used by pregnant women or people who have high blood pressure or heart problems.**

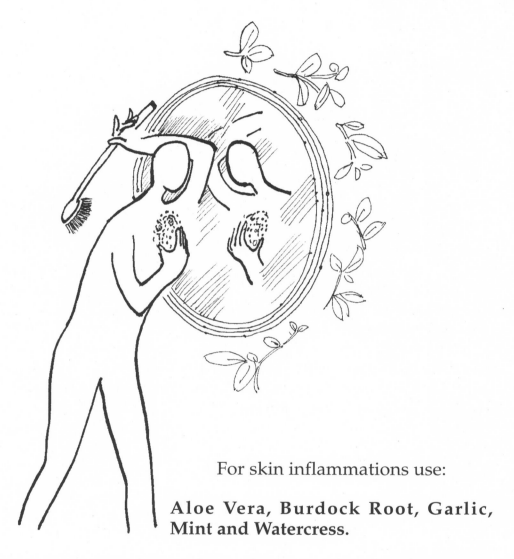

For skin inflammations use:

Aloe Vera, Burdock Root, Garlic, Mint and Watercress.

To encourage sweating and circulation in the skin use: **Basil, Bay Leaf, Cayenne Pepper, Cinnamon, Fresh Ginger Root, Green Onion and (hot) Sage, Thyme**

STIMULATE LUNG FUNCTIONS

Of course, no smoking – of any substances!

BREATHE DEEPLY

Open the lungs wide by throwing the arms open while inhaling deeply through the nose and slowly counting to seven. Then exhale slowly through the mouth while counting to seven and exhaling as you fold your arms across your chest. Repeat three times. Do this deep breathing exercise every day to stimulate lung functions. The best time to do deep breathing exercises is between 6 and 8 am while the air is still fresh.

If your chest is congested or you are coughing, avoid all dairy products. If you live in the city, take monthly trips to green, woodsy high altitudes (over 3 thousand feet elevations) where the air is usually more clear and vitalized than city air.

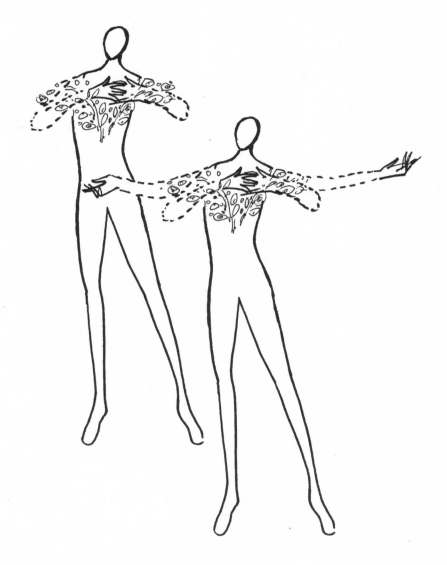

To stimulate lung functions use:

Caraway, Cayenne Pepper, Chives, Cinnamon, Fennel, Fenugreek, Garlic, Horseradish, Marjoram, Mint, Mustard Seed, Onions, Orange Peel, Oregano, Thyme, Watercress

STIMULATE KIDNEY FUNCTIONS

BREATHE DEEPLY

"Charge" the kidneys by raising the arms above the head while inhaling deeply through the nose. Hold the breath and stretch for a few seconds. Then exhale slowly through the mouth as you lower the arms and touch the toes keeping your legs straight. If you cannot touch your toes, bend down and reach as far as you can comfortably while keeping your legs straight. Repeat seven times. Do this exercise every day to stimulate kidney functions.

Reduce animal products, table salt and sugar at least 50%. However, increase the use of natural and highly digestible sodium-rich foods such as Celery, Okra, and liquid aminos (a salt free but sodium-rich Soya Bean extract). Increase water intake 25 to 50%. This reduces the burden on the kidneys so that they can filter wastes from the blood more efficiently.

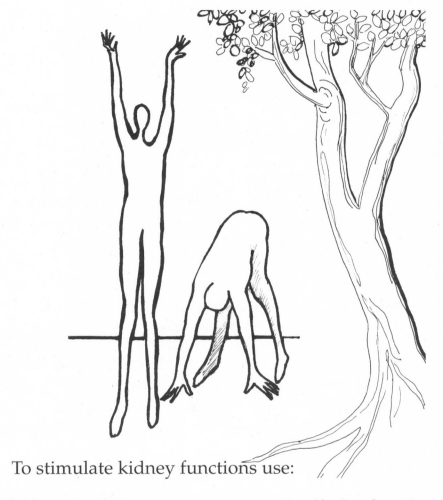

To stimulate kidney functions use:

Alfalfa, Adzuki Beans, Asparagus, Basil, Cardamom, Celery Roots and Seeds, Cloves, Cranberry, Fennel, Fenugreek, Flax Seeds, Grains, Marjoram, Nuts, Parsley, Pomegranate, Sage, Savory, Yucca, Watercress, Watermelon Seeds

STIMULATE LIVER FUNCTIONS

BREATHE DEEPLY

Through the nose, take a huge breath. As the air goes down let it force your lower abdomen to expand. Hold your breath while you make nine great circular motions with the trunk of your body. Exhale through your mouth pressing all of the air out of your abdomen. Repeat three times. This massages your liver and encourages blood circulation.

Fast one day each week. At this time, drink one gallon of distilled water containing the juice of 4 Lemons. The following juices are also helpful: Carrot, Grapefruit, Beet, Celery, Apple and Prune. The average well person can safely extend this fast up to 10 days. Vegetables, vegetarian soups and Grains can be added for more nutrition and energy. One quart of an appropriate herbal tea daily should be included during any fasts. Avoid all animal products, alcohol, caffeine, nuts, sugar, foods containing flour, oils or fats.

CAUTION: Fasting is not advised for pregnant women, diabetics, children under 14 years old or athletes in training.

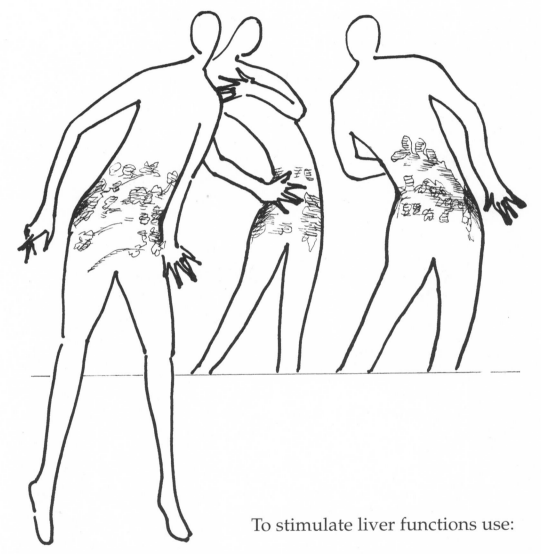

To stimulate liver functions use:

Alfalfa, Aloe Vera, Basil, Burdock Root, Bay, Caraway, Chamomile, Coriander, Dill Seed, Fennel, Flax Seed, "Greens," Lemon, Lemongrass, Rosemary (if the blood pressure is <u>not</u> high), Parsley, Turmeric, Watercress

STIMULATE BOWEL FUNCTIONS

BREATHE DEEPLY

The breathing exercise described on the preceding page is a good beginning for stimulating the colon. In addition, tap the bowel gently from right to left. Repeat 3 times. The combination of deep breathing and massage helps activate movement in the bowel.

Avoid laxatives as they weaken the natural action of the bowels. If you suffer from constipation or sluggish bowels, try the following:

Soak 2 tablespoons of Flax Seeds in 8 ounces of water overnight. Drink in the morning upon rising.

Eat 5 pressed Alfalfa tablets with each meal.

Eat 1/2 cup white or black Bean soup with 1 meal daily.

Eat 1/4 cup Applesauce made with unpeeled, unsweetened Apples.

Eat Cole Slaw or Sprout salads daily. Add 1 tablespoon grated raw Beet Root.

Increase the amount of water you drink.

Two times a year (especially when fasting) have a professional colonic **IF YOU ARE ABSOLUTELY CERTAIN** the Colon Irrigation Therapist uses new, unopened disposable nozzles and tubes. If a colonic is not available, take a one quart enema using a herbal tea made with equal parts: Dandelion, Chamomile and Alfalfa herbs.

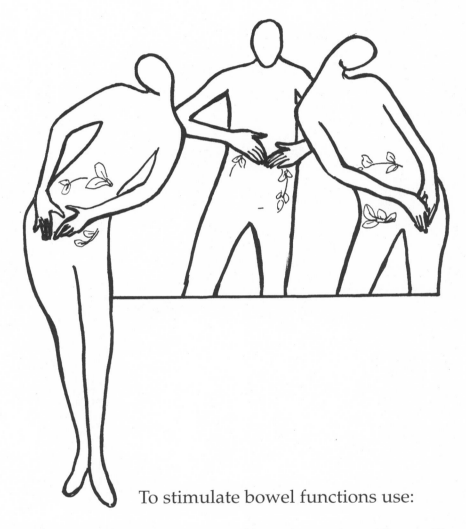

To stimulate bowel functions use:

Agar, Alfalfa, Aloe Vera, Basil, Beans, Beet Root, Burdock Root, Dried Fruits, Flax Seeds, Garlic, Grains, "Greens," Fennel, Fenugreek, Fibrous Fruits, Poppy Seeds, Sesame Seeds, Sprouts, Vegetables, Walnuts

SEVEN

DICTIONARY
OF
COMMON
HOUSEHOLD
HERBS

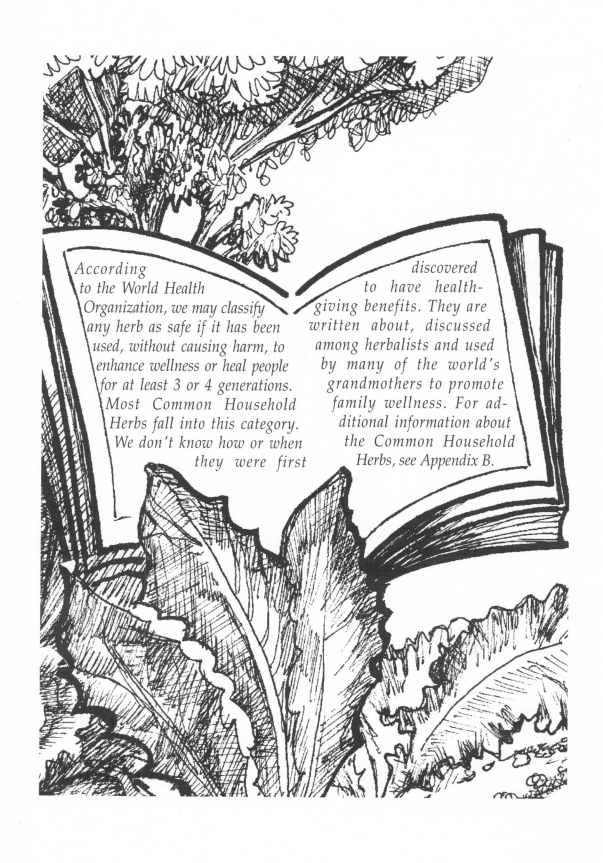

According to the World Health Organization, we may classify any herb as safe if it has been used, without causing harm, to enhance wellness or heal people for at least 3 or 4 generations. Most Common Household Herbs fall into this category. We don't know how or when they were first discovered to have health-giving benefits. They are written about, discussed among herbalists and used by many of the world's grandmothers to promote family wellness. For additional information about the Common Household Herbs, see Appendix B.

AGAR   Is an algae harvested and dried in the sun until it is bleached. It is so rich in minerals that it is used in experimental laboratories as a culture on which to grow living matter. Three heaping tablespoons of Agar flakes or 1 1/2 T powder can be dissolved in 1 pint of water to make a bland tasting, gelatin-like dish. Fruits or vegetables can be added to make a nutritious aspic. It can also be added to blenderized nutritional drinks. Agar is a popular food in many Asian cultures. It is available at healthfood stores or Asian markets.

ALFALFA   Is mineral-rich and can be used as a nutritional supplement. The green substance (chlorophyll) in the leaves is extracted and marketed as a liquid or powdered tonic; it is rich in iron and is, therefore, blood-building. It is also mildly diuretic. When dried and compressed into tablets, Alfalfa is a nutritious, fibrous bulk that can be taken with meals to help cleanse and rejuvenate the bowels. It is a wonderful source of nutrition for nursing mothers. Some say that a cup of Alfalfa tea taken daily over a long period of time is helpful in relieving arthritis pain because it dissolves hard, stony deposits. Alfalfa is one of the few foods containing Vitamin K which helps the blood coagulate in a normal way. Since diabetics frequently experience excess bleeding because their blood coagulates slowly, they would do well to drink Alfalfa tea regularly.

ALLSPICE   Is a warming digestive stimulant.

ALOE VERA   Leaves are succulent. They can be split open and the fresh gelatinous contents applied directly to sores and rashes to stimulate healing. To stop pain, Aloe Vera gel can also be applied to sprains, injuries and burns. Aloe juices can be taken internally to cool inflammations and infections. However, commercially bottled Aloe Vera is not uniform or dependable in therapeutic value. A better way to benefit from this plant is to extract the juice of Aloe Vera leaves in a juicer. Aloe Vera grows wild in desert, savannah and temperate zones. Every household should maintain an Aloe Vera plant to treat burns and injuries. A note of caution: Aloe Vera is internally cooling and should not be consumed by anyone who is experiencing diarrhea and poor digestion due to internal coldness.

ANISE

Stimulates and warms digestion. It helps get rid of gas, belching, abdominal pains and the kind of mucous that develops from poor digestion. Asiatic Indians chew a few roasted Anise seeds after meals to stimulate digestion and sweeten the breath.

BAMBOO SHOOTS

Are the young, sprouting stems of the Bamboo plant – a type of grass. In Chinese medicine, parts of the Bamboo plant are used to reduce mucous and phlegm in the body. This is because the Bamboo plant is "drying." It reduces the water content in the body. It causes water to leave the body via urine, the skin, the lung and the bowel. Being a hot climate plant, it has been given cooling properties to share with humans. Bamboo Shoots are a wonderful summer vegetable that can be added to salads, soups, meat and vegetable dishes. They are especially helpful to diabetics (who tend to retain too much water even though most diabetics experience excessive thirst) as they also slightly reduce blood sugar.

BASIL Primarily relaxes nerves, spasms and tension. Therefore, it calms and aids digestion and helps relieve stress-related headaches and constipation. Because it relaxes muscle spasms, it helps improve circulation. Chinese culture also uses Basil as an antidote for seafood poisoning. Many herbalists include Basil in soothing formulas for individuals who are freeing themselves of drug addictions.

BAY (Laurel) Stimulates digestion and relieves cramping and gas. Bay contains an oil that stimulates circulation when applied to the skin. Therefore, a strong decoction of Bay can be massaged into the limbs of people with circulation difficulties. It can also stimulate hair growth when applied to the scalp. A strong tea made with Bay can help reduce dandruff when massaged into the scalp and wrapped in a towel for one hour before rinsing. A few Bay leaves sprinkled in and around whole grain flours, grains and other herbs discourages pesky little mealy bugs and other parasites from taking over.

BEAN SPROUTS (Lentils, Peas, Mung Beans, Adzuki Beans) Are produced by soaking dried Peas or Beans in water overnight. In the morning strain and rinse them. Keep them moist by rinsing them off 2 times daily. They should be kept in a darkened place until they break open and begin to sprout – 2 or 3 days. Young Sprouts are very rich in vitamins and minerals. They lose much of their starch content and improve their protein quality upon sprouting. After sprouting, they can be placed in the sunlight for a day in order for the leaves to turn green. Every household should store Beans in case of emergencies because Beans can serve as a meat substitute, a starch or, when sprouted, a vegetable. Mature Mung Bean Sprouts (the kind available in markets) have been found to be cooling to people who are internally hot.

BURDOCK ROOT

Is a thin carrot-like root that is used much in Japanese culture where it is called "gobo". It is slightly bitter but, peeled and sliced, it blends well with other vegetables in soups, stir fries and with grains. Burdock Root also grows wild in North America where it has been found rich in magnesium and potassium. Studies by early United States pharmacists and medical doctors frequently discussed using Burdock Root and Seeds to make extracts and powders for treating liver and skin diseases.

CACTUS PADS

Grow wild in the hot, dry climates of Mexico and California. They are very popular in the Mexican diet where they are called "nopales." These flat, succulent pads are covered with thorns that must be removed before they are edible. They contain a thick, sticky juice similar to that found in okra and are prepared in the same way. Cactus Pads taste somewhat like stringbeans and contain a similar chemical activity that stimulates insulin functions.

Some diabetics have reported success in regulating their blood sugar by drinking 1/4 cup of extracted Cactus Pad juice each morning. This same juice can be applied to swollen, painful injuries and joints for relief.

CARAWAY   Aids digestion and eliminates "gas" because of its antacid (1/2 teaspoon) and anti-spasmodic properties which also relieve the spasms of uterine cramps. In nursing mothers it increases the amount of breast milk. When suffering a griping feeling after taking a laxative, a cup of Caraway tea can ease discomfort. And, Caraway often helps to cough up phlegm from congested lungs.

CARDAMOM   Is a carminative. That is, it stimulates the digestive organs and metabolism of fluids. For example, if digestion is sluggish, too much mucous, phlegm and bloating results. This "dampness" may rise upward and congest the upper body. Cardamom assists the digestive processes so that such dampness is decreased. It is sometimes called the "Queen of Spices" because of its efficiency in improving digestion and the availability of nutrients from the food we eat. Ultimately, nerve and brain functions are enhanced by the actions of Cardamom. However, excessive use of this herb can lead to diarrhea, fatigue and decreased interest in sexual activities.

CAYENNE PEPPER   Is also called "Capsicum" and "Red Pepper." When taken moderately, it stimulates and warms digestion. However, its major value is that it

---

stimulates the circulation of blood. Ironically, it also stops bleeding (both internally and when applied externally). When used in herbal formulas, it acts as a carrier for other herbs. Paprika is a less pungent, milder form of Pepper that can be used in larger quantities to garnish and color other foods.

CELERY
Stalks are a wonderful source of dietary fiber and should be added generously to soups, sauces and other dishes. Celery is a good source of highly digestible sodium which is necessary to counteract overly acidic conditions arising from eating too much animal foods. Celery stalks can act as a coolant for people who tend to perspire and dehydrate. Many people have reported eating several Celery stalks or drinking about 2 cups of Celery juice daily to lower blood pressure. Celery roots strengthen the functions of internal organs — probably through an influence on the nervous system. Celery seeds act as a diuretic; they remove excess water while they slightly strengthen kidney, liver and bladder functions. Celery seeds are warming to the body and calm the nerves. Their nutritional value can be extracted by blenderizing them in vegetable juices, plain yogurt, buttermilk, salad dressings and by adding them to soups, vegetables and breads. Because all parts of the Celery plant are rich in sodium, it is strengthening to the stomach (the fluids of which require sodium) and digestion.

CHAMOMILE
Is a tiny flower that grows abundantly in most yards and curbsides. It is usually mistaken for a

weed but early herbalists respected this herb for its ability to relax nerves. This is one reason it is often included in the selection of teas offered at a growing number of restaurants and markets. Many people tend to eat when they are worried and/or stressed. Digestive organs are not able to function well under these circumstances. A cup of Chamomile tea is helpful to relax the nerves so that proper digestion can occur. In fact, Chamomile is so relaxing that a cup of this tea can be taken at bedtime to encourage sleep. Chamomile also stimulates liver functions. When mixed in equal parts with parsley and chervil (an herb used more in French cooking), a tea can be made for an eyewash in cases of eye inflammations. After using the herbs for steeping, the used herbs can be put into cheesecloth and placed over the eyes. This is both restful and healing. However, it is important to first consult an ophthalmologist.

CHIVES Function similar to onions. They provide warming energy for the body. Therefore, they aid digestion and stimulate circulation.

CILANTRO (See CORIANDER.)

CINNAMON Energizes and warms the entire body. It stimulates circulation and digestion and helps rid joints and muscles of stiffness caused by cold weather. After being "caught out in the cold," a cup of Cinnamon tea can help prevent the onset of a head cold. People who suffer from internal coldness, lack of energy and signs of poor digestion, benefit greatly from the warmth and energy of a little Cinnamon added to a spicy herbal tea daily. (The tonic effect can be enhanced by adding a little ginger root.) Cinnamon has been found to have both antiseptic and fungicidal benefits.

CLOVES   Stimulate and warm digestion. They also encourage digestive energy to descend thus preventing nausea and hiccoughs. Cloves are a natural antiseptic. If a Clove is held in a tooth cavity, its natural oils can quell the pain of a toothache and reduce bacteria in the mouth. Therefore, Cloves are a mouth deodorant. Cloves are also a tonic for exhausted kidney energy. (Use only when symptoms indicate internal coldness: loose stools, excess water, chills and low back discomfort.)

CORIANDER   Seeds are warming and aid digestion by strengthening the functions of the stomach, liver and gall bladder. Coriander helps relieve abdominal gas and spasms. One reason curries and masalas benefit digestion is that they contain Coriander powder. The leaves of Coriander are called "Cilantro" and contain many minerals and vitamins that enhance nutrition. They can be added to soups, salads and sauces to enhance flavor and nutrition.

CORNSILK   Is the silky strands found atop unshucked fresh corn. When dried and made into a tea it clears away fluid retention in people who have a tendency to feel hot internally. Cornsilk, used regularly, helps dissolve hard deposits in the body (i.e., kidney/gallstones). Combine parsley and Cornsilk for a stronger solution. When urination feels hot, stings and is darker and stronger than usual, there may be infection. First seek medical intervention. Secondly, add Cornsilk tea to the daily diet to cool and clear any possible bladder inflammation. (Cranberry extract or juice can be added to this tea for a stronger effect.)

CUMIN Stimulates digestion, increases appetite and eliminates gas. It is often used in making curry and masala powders. Cumin should be used in soups and sauces especially by people who have poor digestion and tend to form lots of mucous. Cumin contains a higher percentage of iron than most herbs.

DILL Leaves are rich in potassium, calcium and sodium. They strengthen digestion and help relieve colic partly because Dill contains a substance that speeds up the formation of enzymes. Therefore, Dill is often used instead of vinegar in the making of brines, sauerkraut and pickles. Dill seeds also promote the flow of milk in nursing mothers (Combine 1 ounce powdered Dill seeds + 1 ounce chamomile + 1 pint rice wine [Saki] in a sealed bottle. Shake daily for 2 weeks. Strain. Take 2 teaspoons 2 times daily.).

FENNEL Leaves and stalks stimulate digestion and increase movement of the bowels (peristalsis). The seeds have anti-spasmodic properties and relieve abdominal spasms (especially if dry roasted). Fennel helps the lungs expel phlegm. Research has found Fennel helpful in "tuning up" the digestion of cancer patients who are undergoing radiology or chemotherapy. Another benefit of Fennel is its ability to clear vision and remove "floaters" that blur vision. Fennel reinforces kidney energy in the same manner as cloves. These two herbs can be used in combination for this purpose. Because it warms and strengthens the lower body, Fennel is effective in regulating chronically late menstrual periods and preventing inguinal hernias (Pour 1 cup boiling water over 1/2 ounce ground Fennel Seeds. Steep 15 minutes. Drink each morning before eating.).

FENUGREEK SEED

Is very popular in India where it is one of the herbs used in making curries and masalas. Traditional Indian physicians (called Ayurvedic doctors) use Fenugreek to relieve lung and throat conditions caused by viruses and bacteria. (Perhaps this is partly due to the fact that Fenugreek contains nicotinic acid which repels and kills parasites and insects.) Ayurvedic doctors soak 2 teaspoons of the seeds in a glass of water for 4 hours. Then, they boil the mixture down to 1/4th of the original volume, strain and add honey. Their patients drink this mixture every night to moisten and improve lung functions. For centuries Ayurvedic doctors have also used Fenugreek to increase the quantity and flow of milk in nursing mothers. Its ability to bring moisture to the upper body makes it helpful to people who suffer from dry throat and excessive thirst. This means that diabetics should use

Fenugreek regularly in soups, stews and sauces. It should be avoided by those congested with mucous and/or phlegm. It is popular among Chinese herbalists who use it in herbal formulas to treat coldness in the lower body and where the "sexual fire is extinguished" by internal coldness. For this purpose, Fenugreek can be used in combination with fennel and cloves.

FLAX SEED   Stimulates efficient bowel elimination by moistening and lubricating the bowel. Flax Seeds can be pulverized easily in a blender and the powder mixed with water into a thick paste to be applied externally to bruises and swellings. This poultice, left on overnight, draws out soreness and abscesses. Juices and oils pressed out of Flax Seeds have been injected rectally to reduce inflammation in hemorrhoids and the prostate gland. Singers can sometimes clear "raspy" throats by soaking a tablespoon of Flax Seeds overnight in 1/2 cup water. Stir and drink this mixture in the morning. Flax Seeds contain oils that nourish the nerves, spinal cord and brain. In fact, Flax Seed oil is reputed to be the only vegetable oil that contains all 3 Omega oils present in fish. These oils are rich in fatty acids essential to human health and the reduction of cholesterol. However, for maximum benefit, Flax Seed oil must be freshly pressed, untreated and unheated.

FRUITS
(Common Fresh)   Each season produces the kinds of fruits humans require for maintaining internal balance. Fresh Fruits are generally cooling. Therefore, they are

more plentiful in the summer when we tend to overheat and need coolants to prevent dehydration (*See Watermelon*). Fresh Fruits often cause gas when eaten along with vegetables. It is better not to mix the two. Cold natured people who tend to retain water and have loose and/or runny stools should not eat an excess of juicy fruits — especially when the weather is not hot. Many fruits contain specific healing chemical activity:

Avocado Seeds soaked in rubbing alcohol or vinegar for 3 months makes a liniment that is sometimes helpful in reducing pain in aching arthritic joints.

Cherries help to lower gout-causing uric acid levels in the blood. Cherries are also blood-building.

Citrus Fruits (Oranges, Tangerines, Grapefruits, Lemons, Limes) stimulate the body's internal "cleansing" processes. In Chinese medicine one to eight year old dried Tangerine or Orange Peels are used to dislodge and remove phlegm. Citrus fruits and beverages should be consumed in the mornings so that they have the entire day to work their cleansing action on the body. (Vegetables should be taken in the evening because they neutralize acids created during the day.) Since people over 40 are entering the biological stage of "demineralization" (otherwise known as "aging" or breaking down), they should limit the intake of citrus foods and increase consumption of mineral-rich herbs. Recent findings reveal Grapefruit seeds contain a powerful anti-fungal, anti-bacterial substance that is now extracted for commercial use. Three drops of this extract in 4 ounces of water serves as a mouthwash, douche solution or disinfectant.

Coconuts are very nourishing – especially to very young children, elders and those who are dehydrated from fevers and illness. In this case, cut the top off a green, tender Coconut and drink all the juice daily. A tablespoon of honey added enhances the tonic effect. For even greater nutritional value, blend the water and soft fresh Coconut meat together. (The soft meat is easier to digest than dry, hard Coconut because it contains less fat.) Both tender and dry Coconut meats can be pulverized and applied to all types of skin problems. And Coconut Oil serves as a good base for making herbal salves, ointments and hair preparations.

Cranberries are sometimes useful in clearing kidney and bladder inflammation. However, they contain oxalic acid (as does rhubarb, cooked spinach and chard) which can irritate joints and cause stone formation when eaten excessively. Therefore, Cranberry juice should not be consumed routinely as a "refreshing beverage." It's actually a medicine.

Dry Fruits are mineral-rich. Dried figs are one of the highest sources of potassium. Two Black Mission Figs each morning help reduce nasal mucous. Prunes not only stimulate bowel function but contain nerve-building chemicals. Dried Apricots are rich in vitamin A, iron and copper; they help build blood and stimulate liver functions. However, dried Fruits are highly concentrated in sugars. Therefore, they should be eaten in very small quantities.

Grapes and all parts of the Grape plant target their benefits to the liver. The acids in Grapes help the liver's detoxification functions. The juice is cooling and thirst quenching. The leaves added to the diet and/or made into a tea help remove damp and oily rashes from the skin. The iron content of Grapes helps build blood. Grape seeds contain oils that have been found helpful in regulating hormonal activity, strengthening the body's immune responses and increasing the strength and flexibility of blood vessels throughout the body.

Lemon stimulates the liver's detoxifying functions. It can be diluted with water (25 parts water to 1 part lemon juice) while on internal cleansing fasts. Or, taken as a morning tea to "get the body" (including the bowels) started. Although it is acidic in nature, its function is to alkalinize the body. Its flavor resembles salt making it a good salt substitute.

Loquats impressively lower blood pressure in an emergency. However, they cause the body to retain water so that people with asthma or excess mucous should not eat them. The leaves of the Loquat tree are used by herbalists in several cultures to stop coughs caused by dry lungs and throat.

Melons are very moistening to the internal body; they should be eaten abundantly by those suffering dehydration and internal heat – especially in the summertime. In addition, Cantaloupe, being an orange colored food, is rich in vitamin A, a vitamin now recognized to be essential in fighting cancer. (See Watermelon Seeds)

Persimmons are moistening to the lungs and bowels and so help with dry coughs where there is also constipation. But they should not be used by those with asthma and/or loose bowels.

Pineapple has a positive impact on the immune system. When antibiotics are taken with Pineapple juice, the benefit of the medication is greater. Pineapple can be made into a paste and used on wounds (including dental surgery) to reduce swelling and inflammation. It helps to destroy fungus; therefore, athlete's foot and toenail fungi often get better when soaked in blenderized fresh Pineapple 1 hour daily. Pineapple causes a slight thinning of the blood. It should be used by those who need this function. However, it should be avoided by those who have a tendency to bleed easily.

Pomegranates encourage the production of female hormones in menopausal women. It is sometimes added to herbal formulas to take the place of estrogen. Since female hormones are sometimes used in treating male prostate and sexual problems. Pomegranates are useful to some "menopausal" men. Pomegranates contain oxalic acid and should not be used excessively.

Tomatoes originated in Native American culture where they were considered a medicine. Since they are juicy and cooling, they were traditionally used for dry coughs and in hot weather.

Tropical Fruits such as Papaya, Mango and Pineapple contain enzymes that help digest proteins. In tropical countries, they are eaten along with meats for this purpose. Papaya should be avoided by people who are taking anticoagulants because it encourages blood to coagulate.

GARLIC   Is one of the great herbal panaceas. First, it is rich in sulphur which accounts for some of its antibacterial strength. It helps decongest and resolve inflammation throughout the body. For example, mildly inflamed hemorrhoids will shrink if a large clove of Garlic is peeled, cut open and inserted into the rectum overnight. (Do not be discouraged by its medicinal action causing a harmless burning sensation.) Congested lungs may also be cleared by eating several cloves of fresh Garlic or a daily dose of dried, deodorized Garlic capsules. For some people, digestion is improved by taking Garlic capsules with meals. Blood pressure and circulation can often be normalized by taking from 3 to 9 Garlic capsules daily. Intestinal parasites seem to detest Garlic. Intestinal worms can sometimes be driven out of humans and animals by consuming large amounts of Garlic. Recent scientific investigations confirm the fact that Garlic plays a role in preventing cancer.

GINGER

Is one of the most pungent and warming herbs. When taken dry, Ginger warms the stomach and intestines thereby stimulating digestion and relieving abdominal spasms caused by internal coldness. Fresh Ginger, taken as a tea, is particularly warming to the surface of the body thus encouraging sweating. It is very helpful during the first stages of chills at the onset of a "cold." In general, Ginger is helpful in stopping nausea, vomiting and loose bowels caused by weak digestion. A cup of Ginger tea helps resolve morning and motion sickness. Asian people often eat a mealtime condiment of sliced Ginger preserved in either salt or sugar and vinegar. This helps stimulate and strengthen digestion. When consuming slightly toxic herbs/foods, a cup of Ginger tea may act as an antidote.

GRAINS   And grain-like grasses (i.e., unrefined Wheat, Buckwheat, Rice, Oats, Millet, Rye, Barley, Quinoa, Amaranth, Corn) are rich in vitamins and minerals and are very important in supporting the functions of the immune, digestive and nervous systems. When mixed with either seeds (sesame, sunflower, poppy, pumpkin, etc.), beans, dairy products or seaweeds, Grains form a high quality protein that can substitute for meats. The fiber in Grains help protect the body from some of the damages caused by pollutants and pesticides. The digestibility and energy-giving aspects of Grains are increased if the Grains are slightly browned in a dry pan before they are cooked with water. Nourishing Grain teas can be made from these "roasted" Grains. Use instead of coffee. 1 cup mixed uncooked Grain can be chopped finely in the blender and cooked in a quart thermos. Fill the thermos with boiling water, close and leave several hours. Use at mealtime. To improve the digestibility and increase the protein value of Grains, they should be sprouted 2 days before using.

Amaranth originated in the Aztec civilization and has only recently found its way into the United States culture. Amaranth is almost as rich in iron as Quinoa. One half cup of Amaranth contains the same amount of calcium as 1/2 cup milk and 95% of our daily magnesium requirement. It forms a complete meat substitute when mixed with either Wheat, Rice or Barley.

Barley is used in Chinese medicine as a cooling diuretic. That is, it helps remove "swamp-like" (hot, damp sediment) conditions such as male/female yellow discharges. It is also effective in cases of excess phlegm and congestion that has settled in the middle and/or lower body. Because the hull is difficult to digest, it is sometimes dehulled and called "Pearl Barley." Since it is almost gluten-free, it does not create the same digestive and allergic reactions as Wheat. It is also very rich in potassium which helps to reduce the acid content of the blood.

Buckwheat is an internally warming grain, rich in nutrients that nourish the heart and blood vessels.

Corn is a vegetable when it is fresh and ripe. However, when it dries, it is classified as a grain. Much of the great nutritional value of Corn is in the germ. Therefore, it should not be refined. It is starchy thus cornstarch is made from it. Corn matures in the summer making it a cooling grain.

Millet is a very light, mild and nutritious grain that restores the strength and is well tolerated by sick people who have lost their appetite. It contains less fat and fewer calories per cup than other grains. Millet is the only grain that is alkalinizing thus it is an ideal grain for meat eaters and diabetics who tend to form excess acid. In many East African communities, Millet gruel is fermented into an intoxicating but highly nourishing traditional beer.

Oats contain a high fat content that lubricates the bowels and helps lower cholesterol. Since Oat flour does not contain gluten, it is not as effective for baking as wheat. Oats are the primary ingredient in most granolas. And they are very nourishing to the nervous system. Oats can be boiled in water, strained and the water used to bathe skin problems on the face or body.

Quinoa is a super-grain. Although it was an important staple of the Inca civilization, it has only recently been "discovered" in United States culture. Quinoa contains more nutrients than any other grain and is the only grain with a protein content so complete that it does not need to be mixed with any other food to take the place of meat. One half cup of Quinoa supplies 60% of a day's iron requirement.

Rice is the grain highest in starch (energy-giving) and low in protein and fat content. It is sweet, heavy and strengthens the digestive system. The polishings (outsides) of Rice grains are very rich in B complex vitamins. Rice cooked into a gruel or porridge is very nutritious for children or people recovering from illness. Wild Rice has a higher mineral content than brown Rice. And white Rice is very low in nutritional value. Although Rice provides much energy by virtue of its starch content, it does not build the muscle mass that protein-rich Wheat and Rye build. Rice can be made into a gruel, like oatmeal, and eaten to correct diarrhea.

Rye originated in Asia but came to the United States as a weed that mixed itself into Wheat and Barley fields. It has never become as popular in the United States as it did in Europe. It is less fatty and has fewer calories than Wheat but equals these grains in building muscle mass and energy. Rye does not aggravate allergies as does Wheat.

Wheat is rich in protein because of its gluten content. Gluten is what permits Wheat flour to expand when it is baked. Gluten is also a highly allergic factor. People with asthma and allergies often improve when they stop eating Wheat products (breads, pastas, crackers and pastries). Pastry flours have more Gluten added to create a "light" texture.

"GREENS" (Collards, Mustards, Turnip Tops, Kale, Dandelions) Are mineral-rich, cooling and alkalinizing. They (especially Dandelion) help prevent inflammations partly because of their high sulphur, iron and vitamin A contents. Collards however, tend to be a little too coarse for the delicate linings of the digestive tract. They should be eaten sparingly or mixed with softer Greens. Greens are an ideal food for activating sluggish bowels. They are a perfect milk replacement for those who can't tolerate dairy products. One cup of Greens (especially Kale) contains calcium equal to one cup of milk. Greens have additional value in that they also contain high levels of iron, magnesium, potassium and vitamin A. (Spinach, Chard and Beet tops are also highly nutritious but contain high amounts of oxalic acid which interfere with the body's ability to utilize its calcium supplies.)

HORSERADISH Is a pungent, warming and stimulating herb that helps digestion and circulation. When grated fresh and mixed with other foods in very small quantities, Horseradish helps relieve rheumatic complaints in some people. Make a massage oil by grating some of the fresh root in olive or sesame oils. Let stand in direct sunlight for 2 days before straining and using. It has antibacterial qualities similar to garlic. Even when commercially prepared, Horseradish is a helpful condiment for people who are burdened with phlegm, sinus congestion and poor digestion.

LEGUMES   Are pods containing seeds such as Adzuki Beans, Black Beans, Black Eyed Peas, Carob*, Garbanzo Beans (Chick Peas), Lentils, Mung Beans, Navy Beans, Peanuts**, Soya Beans***, Yellow and Green Peas. Beans are an excellent meat (protein) substitute if they are accompanied by seeds, grains or dairy to complete their deficient protein content. Excess Beans are not suggested for people who tend to form kidney stones because they may aggravate this condition. Beans are very starchy and difficult for many to digest – explaining why they cause "gas" for most people. Therefore, Beans should be cooked with herbs (listed in this section) that enhance digestion, eliminate "gas" and prevent the formation of stones. They may also be pre-soaked and sprouted to improve their digestibility. And some people have found that freezing beans before cooking decreases "gas" formation during digestion.

*Carob (*also called St. John's Bread*) is a chocolate colored pod that grows on trees in temperate climates. The entire pod is powdered and marketed as a chocolate substitute. It is rich in calcium, naturally sweet and high in fiber. It does not contain oxalic acid, caffeine or cause allergic reactions as does chocolate. Carob can be used to stop diarrhea. It is mild and nutritious; therefore, it is good for children and infants — a teaspoon of the powder can be added to their food or milk.

Peanuts *(also called Groundnuts)* are actually beans. In some areas of the U.S., they are boiled and eaten soft. In Chinese culture, boiled, mashed peanuts are used to increase breast milk in nursing mothers. In the West, some physicians recommend diabetic patients eat a few raw peanuts before meals to temporarily lower blood sugar levels and decrease the appetite. Peanuts contain a higher quality protein, more B vitamins (especially niacin) and dietary fiber than all nuts. However, they are 50% fat, and should not be eaten by people who are overweight. Excessive use of Peanuts also causes a high level of acidity. Caution should be taken in selecting Peanuts as they are a primary source of aflatoxin, a mold that grows on Peanuts and causes liver cancer if consumed in large amounts. Avoid Peanuts that seem moldy or irregular in color or texture. Since heat tends to destroy this mold, dry roasted Peanuts may be safer than raw Peanuts.

***Soya Beans** contain the closest protein quality to meat making it a good meat substitute. Most imitation meat and dairy products such as "textured" protein products, Soya milk, Soya cheese and Tofu are made from processed Soya. Soya is classified as an internally cooling food. Legumes are difficult to digest. Therefore, Soya milk substitutes should be replaced by seed and nut milks *(see Recipes)* for infant formulas.

LEMONGRASS Is rich in vitamin A and anti-viral properties making it a protector against flu viruses and infections. Traditionally, some cultures in West Africa use a morning cup of Lemongrass tea to prevent colds. Thai culture uses whole Lemongrass leaves to give soups and stews a delicious lemon flavor. Mexican culture mixes Lemongrass with hibiscus flower to make a tart but tasty beverage.

MARJORAM Is sometimes called "Woman's Herb" because, once it gets into the body, it gravitates toward the uterus (to bring on delayed menses), the heart (to calm it), the brain and nervous system (to relax tense nerves). However, men also benefit from the use of Marjoram because it relaxes nerves and spasms. It also stimulates digestion and warms lungs that have been invaded by cold air – from both out-of-doors or air-conditioning.

MINT Is a cooling herb. It helps resolve headaches caused by overheating in the head area — perhaps from over-exposure to the sun, a fever or drafts from hot winds such as the Santa Anas. Mint is also useful in the early stages of a warm-weather cold when the eyes are burning and the throat is scratchy. It is often used as an after dinner tea because it stimulates digestion and relaxes and calms the nerves. Mint oil is used in many toothpastes and liniments because it stimulates blood circulation when applied to the skin.

MUSHROOMS Are actually a fungus. There are many kinds but most of the Mushrooms that grow wild in grasses, fields and forests are poisonous and should not be eaten. Some nutritionists have observed that the Mushrooms we buy in the supermarket have a slight diuretic action but little food value. It is only the Shiitake and Ganoderma (Reishi) Mushrooms that have been discovered to contain anti-cancer, anti-tumor substances and interferon. There is a growing body of research showing that people with AIDS, cancer and tumors experience increases in wellbeing and heightened immune responses while taking Shiitake and/or Ganoderma Mushrooms (usually in capsule form) regularly. Dried Shiitake Mushrooms can be found in bulk at most Chinese herb and produce stores. They can be used in place of common Mushrooms by soaking them in water for an hour and removing their stems before using them for cooking.

MUSTARD SEEDS

Are commercially powdered or mashed and mixed with vinegar, wine and other spices to make a condiment that aids in the digestion of fats. Mustard, like horseradish, is pungent and causes phlegm to leave the lungs and sinuses. Mustard Seed powder can also be made into a paste and used as a poultice or plaster on the chest to decongest the lungs. (Mix together 1 tablespoon each: dry ginger, dry Mustard, salt, and turpentine. Add 3 tablespoons of a hardened fat such as lard. Mix well and spread onto a soft cloth. Apply to the chest. This is safe for all ages and may be left on overnight. It can also be used on arthritic and painful joints if the arthritis is caused or made worse by cold, damp weather.) Mustard Seed Oil can be mixed with rubbing alcohol and used as a liniment. However, Mustard Seed should not be used on joints that are hot and swollen as is the case with most rheumatoid arthritis and multiple sclerosis sufferers.

NUTMEG   Astringes or restrains body fluids that are "pouring downward" causing loose bowels because the "middle" (digestive organs) is too weak to hold the fluids up. While astringing (holding up) this dampness, Nutmeg also strengthens digestion so that gas is eliminated and bowels are firmed up. However, Nutmeg is toxic and causes mental confusion if used in large amounts. It should be used only in the amount of a "pinch" along with safer herbs that have similar functions. (Mace is actually the outside shavings of the Nutmeg seed. Mace has a stronger flavor and is used in the same manner as Nutmeg.)

NUTS   (Almonds, Walnuts, Filberts or Hazelnuts) Are rich in oils essential to efficient body function. They also contain high levels of vitamin E. The above Nuts stimulate kidney and brain functions. However, they contain such a high percentage of fats that one should not eat over 2 ounces at any meal. Pecans, Brazil and Macadamia Nuts are particularly high in fat. Cashews have a higher content of oxalic acid which aggravates high cholesterol and stone formations. Many cultures caution against Cashews. Almonds are, perhaps the most digestible and nutritive of all Nuts. Chinese herbal tradition considers small amounts of Walnuts occasionally to be a kidney and brain tonic and bowel lubricant.

ONION   Is a strong anti-bacterial partly because it is rich in sulphur. Onions are pungent and, therefore, have an affinity for the respiratory system (lungs and nose) and the skin; it clears congestion and phlegm from the lungs. To heighten this function and stop coughs, slice 2 Onions and cover with honey and the juice of a lemon. Cover and let stand for several days. Strain and bottle. Use as a cough syrup or decongestant. This is a particularly mild, safe cough syrup for children. Green Onions warm and stimulate circulation in the skin. So, on cold days, a hot bowl of Onion, chicken, vegetable or miso broth with chopped Green Onions and fresh grated ginger root can help prevent cold air from penetrating the (warmed) skin. Onions also stimulate digestive functions which may explain their worldwide popularity as a seasoning.

ORANGE PEELS   (Dried, thin skinned) Help dissolve mucous from the lungs and digestive organs. They also act as a digestive tonic. People who have access to homegrown or untreated Orange or Tangerine trees can save and dry peelings with which to make a tea after the peels have aged one or more years. The older the peelings, the more medicinal they become.

OREGANO   Has similar functions to Marjoram.

PARSLEY   Is one of the most mineral-rich herbs. It is especially helpful in building blood because of its iron and copper content. It is one of the few herbs that contain many of the B vitamins and is one of the richest sources of vitamin A. The entire herb is medicinal. The leaf stimulates liver and kidney functions. Its rich chlorophyll content sweetens the breath. Parsley root is a diuretic, ridding the body of excess water or dampness. Both the leaf and root help dissolve stone-causing acids. A daily cup of Parsley tea should be taken as a preventive by people who have a tendency to form gall or kidney stones. The stems can be simmered into a tea to release congestive fluids from the chest area. When nursing mothers want to "dry up" their breast milk, they can drink an abundance of Parsley tea.

POPPY SEEDS Taken one hour before bedtime with milk encourage sleep. The oil contained in these seeds help lubricate the bowel to correct constipation. Poppy Seeds also contain a chemical substance that, when made into a seed milk and mixed with sugar, helps relieve dysentery. Poppy Seeds are mildly narcotic. Therefore, they have been known to cause a positive drug test result in some athletes who have eaten foods containing Poppy Seeds.

PUMPKIN SEEDS Help control intestinal (tape and round) worms that many people have without being aware. One tablespoon raw Pumpkin Seeds every morning on an empty stomach is a good intestinal parasite preventive. This daily habit also reinforces glandular/hormonal functions and helps prevent congestion in the prostate gland. This is a preventive measure only. After the onset of these conditions additional approaches are necessary.

ROSEMARY Has an affinity for both the head and liver areas. Its camphor content causes its health giving properties to rise upward "opening the senses" and clearing phlegm from the head so that alertness increases and depression is often lifted.

Nerve and brain functions, vision and blood circulation in the upper body are stimulated by Rosemary. For this reason, it has historically been used by herbalists to increase memory and relieve headaches. It should not be used by those with a tendency for high blood pressure because it causes pressure to rise. Otherwise, Rosemary can be used as a general tonic particularly revitalizing to older people and those with low blood pressure. It has been found to have anti-oxidant properties which help the body neutralize harmful toxins. Rosemary and sage tea make a restorative and stimulating hair rinse for people with dark hair.

SAFFRON   Is most valuable for its ability to stimulate circulation throughout the body. When used with other herbs, it carries them more aggressively throughout the body or to the place for which they have the greatest affinity. Saffron is so powerful that in large amounts it can cause hemorrhages. Because it is very expensive, it is often replaced with MEXICAN SAFFLOWER which has a similar function but is less expensive.

SAGE   Is one of the greatest of all tonic herbs — especially helpful for older people because it revitalizes the nervous, glandular and immune systems. A room temperature cup of Sage tea should be taken 2 times daily for these purposes. (When it is hot, it causes sweating.) Sage also helps promote the menses and strengthens hormone production in menopausal women. It stimulates nerve and brain functions as does rosemary without causing a rise in blood pressure. Sage is a natural antiseptic. Taken internally, it helps reduce inflammations. Used as an external wash on wounds it prevents infections. The seeds of Sage are called ``Chia Seeds'' and are highly nutritious. They were used traditionally by Native Americans to sustain their health and vitality during long fasts. They can also be sprouted and used in salads.

SAVORY　　Is one of the most versatile of all tonic herbs. It stimulates the brain, nerves, glands and digestive functions. It strengthens the immune system and helps prevent infections and fungi from overtaking the body. Savory functions similar to Basil but has a stronger antibacterial and anti-fungal influence. Even though Savory increases physical vitality and energy, it does not create internal heat and dehydration as would Korean ginseng or cinnamon. In fact, Savory helps quench thirst; therefore, diabetics who are frequently thirsty might benefit from a habit of drinking Savory tea or using it regularly as a seasoning.

SEAWEEDS　　(Dulse, Kelp, Kombo, Nori, etc.) Are the most mineral-rich of all herbs. They are also rich in iodine which stimulates the thyroid gland and energy levels. Certain toxins and heavy metals are cancelled out by taking Seaweed tablets daily. These tablets are so concentrated in minerals they can be taken as a mineral supplement. They are usually reasonably priced at health food stores. However, those with high blood pressure should use Seaweed tablets with caution because Seaweed is rich in sodium.

SESAME SEEDS Have the highest fat content of all seeds (2 quarts of oil can be pressed from 9 pounds of Sesame Seeds). These fats however, play essential roles in human nutrition. Sesame Seeds are rich also in calcium, phosphorus, Vitamin E, Lecithin and high quality protein. This makes it very suitable to use as a milk substitute for infants: 1/4 cup Sesame Seeds to 2 cups water. Soak overnight. Blend 1 1/2 minutes then strain. White Sesame Seeds are a popular staple food in the Middle East where soldiers traditionally subsisted on them when no other food was available. Now, they are used abundantly in Halva, Tahini and Hummus. In Chinese culture, Black Sesame Seeds are preferred for their superior nutritional value. They strengthen kidneys, liver and glandular functions. They also help build blood, lubricate the bowels to prevent constipation and increase the energy level. Since Black Sesame Seeds increase the underpinning of the human body, older people should add them to soups, sauces and herbal tonics to help reverse the aging process. Sesame Oil is considered the most stable of all oils; it does not become rancid easily and it does not break down quickly when heated. Asiatic Indians have found it the best oil with which to massage the body because its properties are absorbed through the skin. It is used abundantly in Asiatic Indian cooking because of its stability and nutritional value. CAUTION: In general, overweight people should avoid dietary fats and most oils because of their high caloric levels. However small amounts of fatty acids are required for good health. Sesame, flax and olive oils are considered the best sources of these fatty acids. They should be taken in their freshly pressed, unprocessed form and should not be heated to frying temperatures. (Flax Seed oil should not be heated at all.)

SUNFLOWER   Seeds contain nutritional and medicinal value similar to that of sesame seeds but Sunflower Seeds contain an additional amount of A and B vitamins and it is one of the few plant sources containing vitamin D. In Asiatic Indian culture, pulverized Sunflower Seeds are used as a remedy for throat irritation, cough and flu. Chinese herbalists suggest mixing Sunflower Seeds with celery juice to lower blood pressure. The leaves can be made into a tea to reduce viral fever. The petals may be steeped in case of bronchitis. Sunflower Seeds sprout into delicious greens.

TARO ROOT   Is a potato-like tuber found in the produce department of most large markets that serve Asian, Pacific Asian, African, Caribbean and the Southerly American populations. In the Hawaiian Islands it is the main staple food called "poi." It is no coincidence that Taro is the chosen staple of a people who live in a hot, damp climate. These are the very conditions herbalists of other cultures treat with Taro Root. In Japan Albi (Taro) plasters are used to normalize swollen glands and inflammations. A paste is made of 40% white flour, 10% dry powdered ginger root and 50% Taro Root flour. Add water and mix into a paste. It is then applied to affected areas, covered with a damp cloth, wrapped securely and left on for several hours. These plasters are applied daily to cysts, inflammations and swollen glands. In many Chinese restaurants, Taro is served in "hot pot" casseroles.

TARRAGON   Stimulates digestion and appetite. It also helps remove phlegm and dampness in those who retain fluids. Many people report enhanced sleep when Tarragon tea is taken just before bedtime.

THYME   Is a lung tonic, strengthening the lungs and immune system so that there is greater resistance to colds and relief from coughing and congestion. For those who are stressed by continual cold and flu symptoms, Thyme mixed with other tonic herbs can help in the recovery from a state of exhaustion.

TURMERIC   Targets the abdominal area where it stimulates the digestive processes and subsequent circulation of blood into the joints, muscles, pelvic and shoulder areas. It prevents food from "just sitting" in the upper digestive organs creating gas, congestion and discomfort. Turmeric can be used as a paste (mixed with pineapple juice or coconut oil) on wet skin conditions. It is mild and can be used on babies with diaper rashes. It's deep yellow adds color to foods. Recently, a chemical ingredient in Turmeric (curcumin) has been found to be an anti-inflammatory and to have a slight impact on the way HIV replicates.

WATERCRESS   Is a mineral-rich tonic herb that may be used as a nutritional supplement. Watercress enhances the functions of glands, nerves and lungs. It encourages blood building and helps neutralize acids created by the over-consumption of meats, other high protein and sugar-containing foods. Fresh Watercress blended with water has been known to be effective as a skin pack or skin wash on damp, itchy skin conditions.

WATERMELON SEEDS Are a diuretic. A teaspoon of dried seeds can be boiled in 1 cup of water and used to "flush" the kidneys so they will more efficiently maintain proper water balance in the body. Watermelon Seeds are used by Middle Eastern cultures in the same way sunflower seeds are used in the United States. The shells are cracked and the kernels patiently removed to "munch" on. Fresh seeds can be dried and saved until they are needed. WATERMELON FRUIT is cooling. Therefore, it is helpful in resolving internal heat problems brought on by summer heat. It should not be used by those who have diarrhea or loose bowels from weak digestion as it may make these conditions worse.

VEGETABLES (Common Fresh) Are good sources of vitamins and minerals. Dark green, yellow, orange and red vegetables are rich in beta-carotene which is necessary in forming the anti-cancer vitamin A. Also known to help prevent cancer are Broccoli, Cabbage, Cauliflower and Carrots. These vegetables, along with Garlic, Onions, and Turnips, contain sulphur which helps to fight infection. Vegetables rich in magnesium such as fresh Corn, Beans and "Greens" help the body feel cool and relaxed. Many vegetables are rich in alkalinizing potassium such as "Greens," Cabbages, Carrots, Beets, Cauliflower, Squashes, Potato skins, Parsnips and Broccoli. It is important to eat a variety of vegetables because each vegetable has a slightly different nutritional content. In addition, some vegetables contain chemical ingredients that have specific healing benefits:

Arrowroot is a nutritious, starchy, tropical root made into a flour. It makes an easily digested porridge for infants, children and convalescents. It can be used as a thickener for gravies and sauces instead of wheat and cornstarch.

Artichokes contain a chemical that helps reduce cholesterol. They are strengthening to liver functions.

Asparagus dissolves stone-causing uric acids. It increases both urine and bowel activities.

Beets help clear toxins from the liver and build the blood. One tablespoon raw, grated Beet Root daily helps activate the bowels.

Carrots are rich in calcium and beta carotene (vitamin A).

Cucumbers have an astringent quality. The juice can be blended with water and used as a facial cleanser and a freshening vaginal douche – especially appropriate for "yellow" vaginal discharges (Blenderize with equal part plain yogurt. Thin the mixture with water. Inject into the vaginal area and retain as long as possible. Repeat as necessary.)

Kale is one of the vegetables richest in calcium and vitamin A.

Radishes aid in the digestion of starches and fats and help clear mucous. A paste can be made with blenderized Radish Seeds to apply to breasts in which there are cysts or tumors.

YUCCA   (The Bayonet Leaf Yucca tree) Can be seen growing all over the Americas. It is one of the most amazing plants in nature. Every part of this plant can be used in a health-giving manner. Currently, medical botany researchers are in the process of verifying claims that the fresh flowers of the Yucca plant are among the growing number of anti-cancer herbs – without the same side effects that present medications have. Native Americans who use the root of the Bayonet Leaf Yucca as a main dietary starch do not suffer from arthritis. They seem to have lower levels of cholesterol and have less digestive disturbances than those who do not use this food regularly. The juices of the Bayonet Leaf Yucca are now being extracted and sold either as a liquid or made into pills. It is available at most healthfood stores. The roots of this plant can be boiled into a sudsing agent for washing clothes and hair. **The Bayonet Leaf Yucca should not be mistaken for the potato-like tuber of the Yuca Plant -- also called Manioc and Cassava, which is a starchy tuber**. Cassava is sold at many ethnic and super-markets where it is also called "yucca" or "yuca." Tapioca is a form of Cassava. Many people unknowingly have a sensitivity to one of the chemical ingredients in potatoes. They subsequently develop joint stiffness and arthritic symptoms. Cassava is a good substitute for potatoes. However, Cassava is very poor in protein content. CAUTION: The Cassava peeling is very toxic and must be thoroughly removed before it is boiled or steamed like a potato. While boiling, the water should be changed several times to pour off any toxic substance. Cassava (Yuca) can be used in soups, stews or baked after steaming.

EIGHT

THE SCIENCE OF PREPARING COMMON HOUSEHOLD HERBS

RULES FOR USING HOUSEHOLD HERBS

RULE #1

The health-giving properties of most plants are most active between the time their seed sprouts and the time they reach maturity. Use young plants.

RULE #2

The less a plant is heated, the more active its health-giving enzymes remain. Most Herbs should not be boiled excessively. Never use a microwave oven to heat or cook Herbs as microwaves disturb the normal chemical structure of foods and destroy many of their enzymes.

RULE #3

Dried Herbs should usually be used in smaller amounts than fresh Herbs. Although the enzyme action is not as strong in the dried plant, its other nutrients are more densely concentrated.

RULE #4

Never use aluminum, copper, plastic or teflon for cooking. These may alter the natural chemistry of plants or give off toxins during herb preparation. Instead, use glass, ceramic, unchipped porcelain, earthenware or stainless steel. In general cast iron should not be used for preparing Herbs. The metal flakes off into the food. However, it can be used for cooking "greens," stews, soups and beans as it enhances the iron content of these foods.

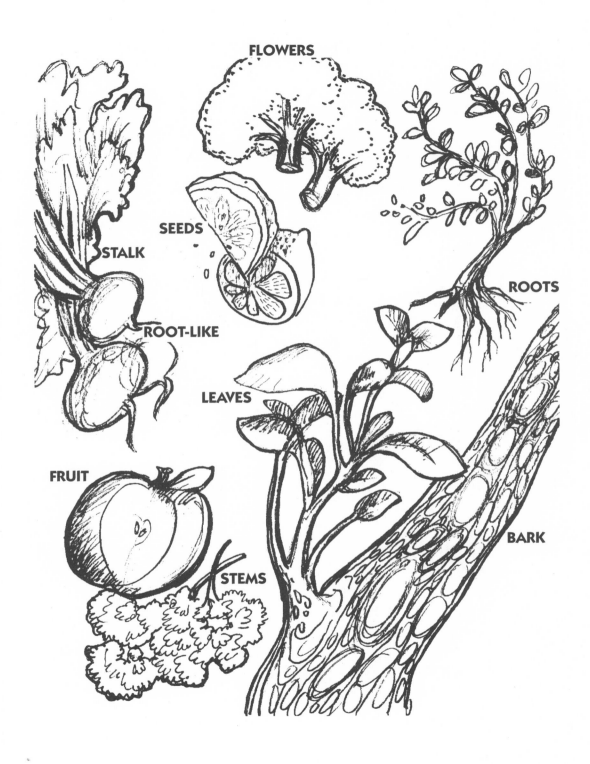

FLOWERS

STALK

SEEDS

ROOT-LIKE

ROOTS

LEAVES

FRUIT

STEMS

BARK

HOW TO PREPARE HERBS

SEES

Seeds are the most vital and nutritious part of the plant. They are the source of new life and usually contain delicate healing oils. Seeds such as Sesame, Flax and Chia should be soaked overnight to soften their outer skin. The mixture can then be blenderized and/or strained before drinking. Dry Seeds can also be powdered in a blender or coffee bean grinder. Add boiling hot water to the powder and let steep 5 to 15 minutes before drinking. Most Seeds can be sprouted. The Sprouts may be eaten raw or made into a tea.

FLOWERS

Cloves, Saffron and Chamomile are delicate Flowers while vegetable Flowers like Broccoli and Cauliflower are more sturdy. Do not boil Flowers. When making teas of delicate Flowers, place 1/2 teaspoon of dry Flowers in a cup and add boiling hot water. Cover and steep 5 minutes. Sturdy vegetable Flowers may be steamed from 5 to 10 minutes in a covered pan.

LEAVES

Mint, Parsley Leaf, Cilantro, Watercress and Alfalfa are tender Leaves that do not require boiling. They can be eaten raw or used to supplement other foods. Tender, spicy Leaves such as fresh Basil, Sage, Marjoram and Rosemary impart their aromas to any foods they are cooked with — even when cooked a long time. However, when leaves are used alone for their medicinal value, they should not be overcooked. Simply pour a cup of boiling hot water over a few fresh leaves (or 1 teaspoon of dried, cut up leaves). Cover and steep 5 minutes before drinking. This is called an herbal "infusion." Tougher leaves such as "Greens," Seaweed, Lemongrass and Bay can be cooked longer to liberate the nutrients from their tough fibers. Leaves can be added to stews, soups or sauces.

STEMS, BARKS and STALKS

Parsley Stems, Celery Stalks and Cinnamon Bark should not be boiled excessively. Cover Stems, Barks and Stalks and simmer about 15 minutes. (Harder barks may need to be simmered longer.)

ROOT-LIKE PLANTS

Some are dense and starchy like Yuca and Potatoes. Others are dense but without a lot of starch content like Carrots, Turnips, fresh Burdock, Parsnips and Beets. Because of their density, they usually need to be cut up and steamed a little longer than flowers and leafy plants.

HARD or DRY ROOTS

Dry Burdock and many other medicinal roots are very tough and hard. To make a tea with dry cut up Roots use approximately 2 ounces of Roots to 1 quart distilled water. Soak for 2 hours. Then cover and boil for 30 minutes. Strain. Simmer the strained tea down to 1 1/2 cups. This concentrated tea is called a "decoction." It is usually stronger than infusions. It can be sipped throughout the day or preserved with 1/4 of its volume in alcohol (vodka or brandy). Shake daily for 14 days. In this alcohol base form, take only 2 tablespoons 3 times daily.

FRUITS

Fruits are most alkaline and sweet at the peak of their maturity. They should be eaten raw in season. While at the peak of their maturity, many Fruits may be dried. Dry Fruits are more dense and, therefore, have more nutritional value than fresh Fruits. Their sugar content is greater, so they should be eaten in small quantities.

USE HERBS IN PURPOSEFUL COMBINATIONS

Herbs in combination are like people in a group. What one person may have difficulty accomplishing alone can be done easier with one or two assistants.

For example, the lungs and sinuses are congested by phlegm rising upward when digestion is incomplete. A combination of Common Household Herbs should be used to both strengthen the middle body and decongest the upper body. Select one to three Common Household Herbs that strengthen digestive (middle body) weakness. Then, select one or two Common Household Herbs that strengthen and decongest the upper body. *(See Chapter Three "To Strengthen Weaknesses")*

Another purposeful combination is formed by using food flavors strategically. In Western culture, not much thought is given to the positive functions of flavors. People are cautioned not to consume excesses of salt because of its effect on kidney functions. Excess sweets are discouraged because they are known to burden the pancreas and liver. But, flavors also have wellness promoting functions.

There are five basic flavors: pungent, sour, sweet, salty and bitter. Taken in moderation pungent flavors such as Ginger, Mustard and Horseradish target and stimulate the lungs; they are decongestants. Sour flavors like Lemons and Vinegar stimulate the liver's detoxifying functions. Sweet flavors of all kinds stimulate and aid digestive organs. Salty flavors such as Celery and Seaweeds cause the kidneys to work harder. And, bitter flavors such as Greens, Beans, Aloes and Burdock tend to break up hardened deposits and "get things going" throughout the body. A well balanced meal should contain each of these five flavors so that the various parts of the internal body will be equally stimulated and balanced.

Every Herb contributes its own unique chemistry to the person who consumes it. In order to maintain a proper internal balance, avoid consuming an excess of particular foods or flavors. Unbalanced food intakes lead to internal imbalances. Combine Common Household Herbs to help balance the flavors and chemistry of your basic diet.

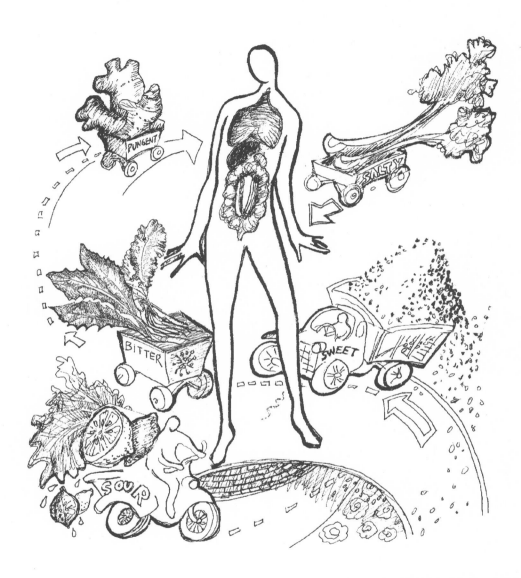

To stimulate all systems of the body in a balanced manner, use the 5 flavors and strengthening Herb combinations to prepare:

Beans, Beverages, Grains, Salads, Salad Dressings, Sauces, Soups, Spreads, Sweets and Vegetable Dishes *(See Recipes)*

NINE

THE ART and SCIENCE PREPARING MEALS WITH COMMON HOUSEHOLD HERBS

THE ART OF PREPARING MEALS WITH COMMON HOUSEHOLD HERBS

Food preparation is an art as well as a science. From a scientific point of view, the person preparing meals should know as much as possible about the general health of whomever food is being prepared for. Scientific knowledge builds a sound basis for the selection of health promoting herbs and other foods.

After selecting the proper foods, an artistic or creative touch should be used to make the foods enticing and delicious to others. This requires using herbs and other foods in new and different ways; not being afraid to experiment.

Use an artistic touch to alter the taste and texture of foods that are disliked. For example, a particular vegetable can be blenderized into a sauce or soup; its taste can be changed by combining it with other Common Household Herbs. Or, it can be finely grated and mixed into a meatloaf or pilaf. With a little creativity, leftovers can be made into new dishes by chopping and using them to fill pastry shells or rolling them in cabbage or grape leaves.

To create such taste thrills without spending half the day in the kitchen, the "cooking artist," like any other artist, must have special tools on hand to work with. The major tools are illustrated on the following page. Other kitchen conveniences that make it easier to create healthy meals quickly are: Rice Cookers, Woks, Juicers, Crock Pots, Dehydrators and Breadmakers.

Time and energy can also be saved by shopping once a week for a week's supply of produce. Refrigerate produce clean by first washing them in a solution of 1 tablespoon Chlorox per 1 gallon water. Rinse thoroughly. Instead of peeling fruits and vegetables, scrub them with a stiff brush. Large quantities of onions and garlic can be chopped and kept frozen till used.

EVERY COOKING ARTIST'S CONVENIENCES

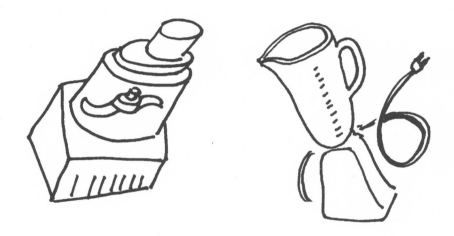

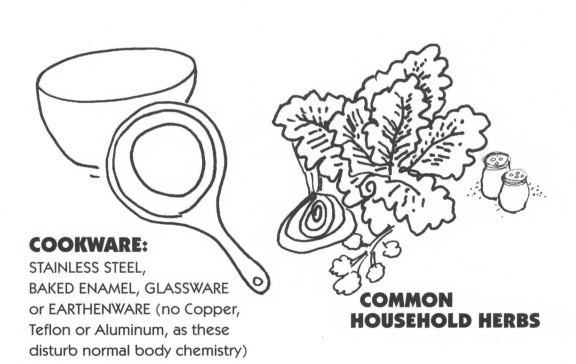

COOKWARE:
STAINLESS STEEL,
BAKED ENAMEL, GLASSWARE
or EARTHENWARE (no Copper,
Teflon or Aluminum, as these
disturb normal body chemistry)

**COMMON
HOUSEHOLD HERBS**

MEAL BUILDING GUIDELINES FOR WELLNESS

A body that does not have existing deficiencies or major imbalances can generally be maintained by a daily intake of the proportions and food categories listed on the following page.

A decision should then be made as to whether the goal of the meal is to reinforce the middle, upper or lower body. If the greatest physical weakness is in the middle body, grains should be dry pan fried till slightly brown before steaming. This cooking procedure will help to strengthen digestion.

If the upper body seems to be the weakest, reinforce the lungs by adding thyme, marjoram and oregano to grains while they are cooking. These herbs also give an appetizing taste and aroma to cooked grain.

If the kidneys or lower area is the most challenged part of the body, seaweed and parsley flakes may be added to grains and vegetables.

At least one meal per day should be based on correcting any internal imbalances that may be present. This can be accomplished by reviewing the information and following the dietary suggestions in *Chapter Four.*

When preparing for an entire family, the special needs of each individual should be met at least twice during a week's period. This can be accomplished best at breakfast and lunch meals. Wellness promoting lunches should be prepared at home and taken to work or school.

While on a detoxification program all meals should exclude foods that may interfere with the elimination of wastes:

ALL Dairy Products and Eggs
Red Meat - Chemically Treated Animal Products
Shell Fish, Catfish, Swordfish, Shark and other Scavengers
Peanuts and Peanut Butter, Yeast Containing Foods
Flour Containing Foods (Bread, Pasta)
Sugar and Sugar Containing Foods
Table Salt, Fried Foods, Chocolate
Black Commercial Tea, Coffee, Alcohol, Sodas and
Fruit Juices (except Lemon, Grapefruit and Prune)

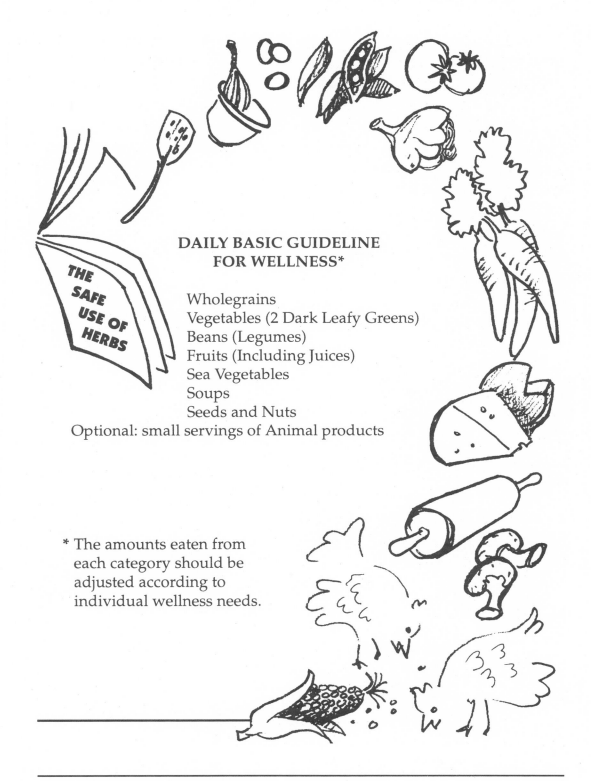

DAILY BASIC GUIDELINE
FOR WELLNESS*

THE
SAFE
USE OF
HERBS

Wholegrains
Vegetables (2 Dark Leafy Greens)
Beans (Legumes)
Fruits (Including Juices)
Sea Vegetables
Soups
Seeds and Nuts
Optional: small servings of Animal products

* The amounts eaten from
each category should be
adjusted according to
individual wellness needs.

TEN

RECIPES FOR WELLNESS

BEVERAGES - ELIXIR MIXERS

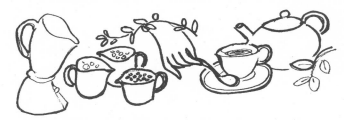

INSTEAD OF COW'S MILK - USE SEED MILK

1/4 cup raw Almonds
1/4 cup Sesame Seeds
1/2 cup Pine Nuts
1 teaspoon Chia Seeds

Soak ingredients overnight in 1 quart of water.
Then blenderize. Strain.
Great for infants, children and adults.
Can use for cooking and on cereals.
Variations:
Sweeten with Date sugar, honey or pure maple syrup.
When used as a children's beverage, add 1 tablespoon liquid chlorophyll for additional iron and minerals.
Add 1/4 cup Coconut milk (from unripe, green Coconut)
Add 1 tablespoon Carob powder for a chocolate flavor.

IF YOU MUST HAVE SODAS - MAKE YOUR OWN

To plain sparkling water add an equal part unsweetened Fruit Juice or 1/8 part of Fruit concentrate.

NUTRITIOUS "SMOOTHY"

2 cups Alfalfa tea
1 tablespoon Agar flakes
1 1/2 cups chopped Fruit(s)
1 tablespoon Sesame Seeds
1 teaspoon Chia Seeds
Honey

To 2 cups boiling water add 2 teaspoons Alfalfa to make a strong tea. Strain and add 1 tablespoon Agar flakes. Dissolve the flakes in the heated tea. Cool and chill. This is the "Smoothy" fluid base. Add remaining ingredients. Blenderize with ice.

PLEASURABLE BUT PURPOSEFUL BEVERAGES

Make an herb tea using a purposeful combination according to need and taste. Use 1/4 cup herb mix to 1 quart boiling water. Cover and simmer 30 minutes. Strain and cool. Add equal part Apple Juice. Keep refrigerated. Drink instead of milk, sodas or pure juices.
Variations:
Use other Fruit juices or Concentrates.

WARM THE MIDDLE GINGER DRINKS

*1 quart fresh honey-
 sweetened Lemonade*
*1/4 cup cut up fresh Ginger
 Root*

Liquefy in blender.
Drink 1/2 cup at mealtime.
Variations:
Use Pineapple Juice instead of Lemon Juice
  Set aside 3 days at room temperature to ferment into a mild wine.

REJUVELAC –
AN ENZYME PROVIDING MILK SUBSTITUTE

1/2 cup rinsed Wheat Grains
1 quart Water

Soak Grains in water for 12 hours. Blenderize and pour into a 1/2 gallon jar. Fill with water and cover. Set aside to ferment for 3 days. Shake daily. Strain and refrigerate. Use as a healthful drink and milk replacement.
Variations:
Add Fruit Juices or Fruit concentrates. Add liquid or powdered chlorophyll to build blood.
Use in place of milk for cooking, baking, dressings and sauces. (However, it adds a sour taste.)

DIGESTION WARMING TEA

2 quarts water
1 teaspoon whole Cloves
4 sticks Cinnamon Bark
8 crushed pods Cardamom
8 thin slices fresh Ginger
    Root
1 piece dried Orange Peel
8 black Peppercorns

Combine ingredients. Bring to a boil. Cover and simmer for one hour. During the last 15 minutes add one ordinary (Black) tea bag. Add 1/2 cup of lowfat milk (if you are not allergic to milk). Sweeten to taste with honey. Drink after meals.
Variations:
Add Fennel Seed and American Ginseng to strengthen the digestion.

EVENING NERVE TONIC

6 oz Carrot Juice
5 Almonds
1 teaspoon Celery Seeds
1 teaspoon Sesame Seeds

Blenderize ingredients.
Variations:
Add 1 tablespoon lecithin granules and 2 tablespoon Rice polishings.
Occasionally add 1 raw egg yolk with 1 Tablespoon Black Cherry concentrate.
(Rice polishings and Black Cherry concentrate are available at most health food stores.)

A CLEANSING JUICE FOR SUMMER FASTING

1 Watermelon

Use 1/2 medium Watermelon daily Remove the outer green skin only (leave the white rind). Cut into small pieces and put fruit, seeds and rind into blender with a little water. Blend until smooth. Drink throughout the day along with water.

IN FROM THE COLD AIR

2 cups of Apple Juice
4 sticks Cinnamon Bark
1 whole Clove
1 teaspoon grated
Ginger Root

Simmer Cinnamon, Cloves and Ginger Root in Apple Juice for 30 minutes. Drink hot.

THE REIGN OF GRAINS

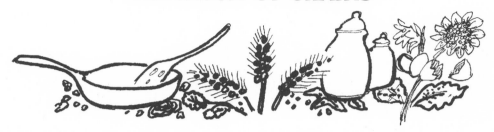

MIXED GRAINS FOR TOTAL NUTRITION

1/2 cup Brown Rice
1/4 cup Wild Rice
1/4 cup Millet
1/4 cup Barley
1/8 cup Quinoa
1/8 cup Amaranth
2 tablespoon Sesame Seeds
1/4 cup Sunflower Seeds

Mix these well. Add water to a level 3 inches over the Grain. Boil till water reaches 1/4 inch above the edge of the Grain. Reduce to a simmer for about an hour. Add more water when Grains become too dry. Takes the place of plain rice.
Variations:
Use a purposeful herbal tea instead of water.

RICE CEREALS FOR NOURISHING CHILDREN OR THE RECOVERING ILL

To cooked Rice stir in enough water to make a smooth gruel (like oatmeal).
Variations:
Add Dates, Raisins and/or Seeds
Use Fennel and Alfalfa Tea instead of plain water.
Mix cooked Rice with cooked Millet.

SPICED RICE

1 cup Rice
2 T Sesame Seed
1 teaspoon Oregano
1 teaspoon Marjoram
1 teaspoon Basil
1 T Sesame Oil

Boil Rice till water is almost gone.
Stir in Sesame Seeds, Oregano, Marjoram, Basil and Sesame Oil.
Variations:
During the last 15 minutes of cooking stir in 1/4 cup Raisins, chopped Dates and/or chopped dry Apricots, 2 T grated Orange Peels, 1/2 teaspoon Cinnamon Powder, 1/2 teaspoon dry Ginger, a pinch of Cardamom and Cloves.

VEGEBURGER PATTIES - A Meat Replacement

1 cup cooked mixed Grains
3 tablespoon fresh chopped
  Parsley
3 tablespoon dry Seaweed
  flakes
1 teaspoon each dry Basil
  and Thyme
1/2 teaspoon each Sage
  and Savory
1 cup cooked Lentils
1 cup chopped Onions
1/2 cup shredded Carrots
1/4 cup sprouted Sunflower
  Seeds

Thoroughly mix ingredients listed. Blend 1 clove Garlic into either 1/2 cup water, Rejuvelac (for a slightly sour taste) or Nut Milk. Mix liquid into dry ingredients. Make into patties and place on cookie sheet. Bake at 400 degrees until brown. Can be frozen and used as needed.

GRANOLA – FOR IMPROVED DIGESTION AND BOWEL FUNCTIONS

3 cups rolled Oats
1 cup chopped Walnuts
1/2 cup Almond slivers
1/2 cup Sunflower and
  Sesame Seed mixture
1 cup chopped Dates
1/4 cup Orange Juice
1 tablespoon Cinnamon
2 tablespoon grated
  Orange Peels

1/2 teaspoon Cloves
2 T Sesame Oil
1/4 cup honey

Separately mix Orange Juice, Cinnamon Powder, teaspoon Cloves, Orange Peels, Sesame Oil and Honey. Combine ingredients and spread in baking pan. Bake one hour at 200 degrees or in a food dehydrator until crisp.

NUTLOAF

1/2 cup chopped Celery
1/3 cup chopped Green
  Pepper
1/2 cup cut up Walnuts
1/2 cup Almond slivers
1 1/4 cups cooked Rice
1 cup Tofu
1 tablespoon Sage
1/2 tablespoon Thyme
1 teaspoon Basil

1/4 cup liquid aminos
1 cup Tomato sauce

Grind nuts together and combine with Rice. Add Tofu and mix. Add other Herbs/Vegetables. Add 1/2 cup of the Tomato sauce and bake for an hour. Uncover and top with remaining Tomato sauce sprinkled with grated cheese. Bake for 10 minutes more. Serve hot.

CORNBREAD PLUS MORE NUTRITION

1/2 cup *Wholewheat flour*
1/4 cup *Millet flour*
1/4 cup *Wheat Germ*
1/2 cup *Wholegrain Cornmeal*
1 tablespoon *baking powder*
1/2 teaspoon *baking soda*
1 cup *either buttermilk or Rejuvelac* (See Beverages)
1/4 cup *Sesame Seeds**
2 *eggs*
1/4 cup *honey* (optional)

Grind in blender.
Shake dry ingredients in a bag. Blenderize liquid with eggs, Sesame Seeds, honey. Mix the ingredients. (More liquid may be necessary.) Bake at 350 degrees for 1 hour or until done.
Variations:
Use 1/2 cup Corn Kernels, 1/4 cup Sunflower Seeds and/or 1 teaspoon dry Herbs of choice.
(Wholegrain Cornmeal available at health food stores) *Sesame Seeds (takes the place of oil)*

PILAF FOR HEALTH AND CREATIVE COOKING

1 large *Onion*
2 *Celery Stalks*
1/2 cup each chopped *Parsley and Celery Leaves*
1 cup shredded *Carrots*
2 1/2 cups *Miso Soup* (See Soups)
1 cup uncooked Rice

Saute ingredients adding uncooked Rice last. Continue to saute until Rice is browned. Separately, make Miso Soup. Add soup to Rice mixture. Cover and simmer for about 45 minutes. When cooked, add 2 cups of chopped Bean, Lentil and Seed Sprouts. (Do not cook further.)

KASHA - A COLD WEATHER WARMER

1 cup parboiled *Buckwheat Groats*
1 cup *Miso Soup*
1 *egg white*

Swish Buckwheat Groats in a bowl containing egg white. Make sure each Grain is coated with egg white. In a dry pan brown the coated Grain till each Grain separates. Add Miso Soup. Cover and simmer till Buckwheat is grainy, soft and tender (about 15 minutes). Use as you would rice.
Variations:
Instead of Miso Soup, use chicken broth or water. More liquid can be used to make this dish a delicious soup. Also add several Green Onions.

WILD RICE SOUFFLE FOR NERVES AND GLANDS

1 cup Wild Rice
1 1/2 cups strained Savory
   and Parsley tea
1 chopped Green Onion
1 chopped Celery Stalk
4 eggs
1 tablespoon Sesame Oil
1 tablespoon Arrowroot or
   Wheat Flour
1/2 cup milk
2 teaspoons finely
   chopped Basil

Simmer Wild Rice in tea mixture. Mix with Green Onion and Celery that have been wilted in 1/3 cup boiling Water.
Separate egg yolks from whites. Beat egg whites till stiff. Set aside.
In a small pan make a cream sauce by mixing Sesame Oil with Arrowroot or Wheat Flour. Slowly add milk and place in a double boiler. Stir until mixture thickens. Slowly add beaten egg yolks and Basil. Combine liquid and Grain mixtures together. Fold in stiffly beaten egg whites. Mix lightly but thoroughly. Pour into casserole dish and place in a pan of hot water. Bake for about 1 1/2 hours at 300 degrees or until set. Serve immediately.

MILLET FOR DIGESTION AND IMMUNE FUNCTIONS

1 cup dry Millet
2 cups water

Cook in the same manner rice is cooked: Boil until water line drops to about 1/4 inch above the Millet. Reduce heat to a simmer. Cover and cook till done - about 30 minutes.
Variations:
Add cooked Beans and Vegetables while cooking.
Make a saute of Onions and other herbs according to need and taste. Mix with cooked Millet and bake at 350 degrees for 30 minutes.
Make a saute of Onions, Celery, Red or Green Peppers. Add a handful of chopped dry Dates and Apricots, 1 tablespoon grated fresh Ginger Root and 1 tablespoon grated Orange Peels. Mix with cooked Millet.

ESPECIALLY PURPOSEFUL VEGETABLES

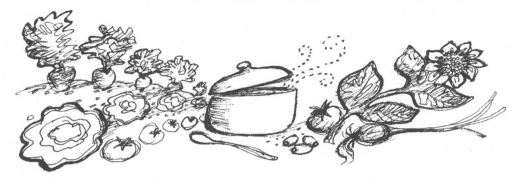

COOLING, CLEANSING, NOURISHING AFRICAN GREENS

1 bunch of Greens*
1 medium Onion
1 small diced Tomato
1 clove finely diced
   Garlic
1 tablespoon Curry
   Powder
Juice of 1/8 Lemon
2 tablespoon liquid
   aminos

*Use Mustards, Turnip Tops,
   Collards, Dandelions,
   Watercress. Mix them or use
   them separately.

Wash and stack Greens flat in a pan. Add 1/2 cup water and wilt by lightly steaming. Cool and cross-cut Greens into small pieces. Set aside.
Saute Onions and Garlic till they are soft and clear. Add remaining ingredients. Simmer 10 minutes. Mix with the cut greens include the nutritious juices. Cover and simmer for 30 to 60 minutes.
Variations:
Use Salsa (See Sauces) on top.
Use any other herbs* desirable.
Place sliced Avocado and/or diced Cucumbers on top.
While saute is cooking add sliced Okra.

ALLEGED CANCER-FIGHTER

Equal parts
Shredded Cabbage
Lightly scraped Grated
   Carrots
Shredded Broccoli Stems
   (skins removed)
Cut up Broccoli Flowers
Sliced Shiitake
   Mushrooms (fresh or
   presoaked dry)

Use only enough water to create steam for 15 minutes. Cover while steaming.
Variations:
Season with other herbs according to need and taste.

TO CLEANSE THE BOWEL

1 cup grated Beet Root
1/2 cup grated Carrot
1/2 Lemon
2 tablespoon of Olive or Flaxseed Oil

Steam Beets and Carrots till softened but slightly crisp. Add the juice of 1/2 Lemon together with Olive or Flaxseed Oil. Mix well.

TO WARM AND DRY THE MIDDLE

20 dry Shiitake Mushrooms
3 cups cut fresh String Beans
2 tablespoon Sesame Oil
4 chopped Green or Red Onions
2 tablespoon dry Tarragon
2 tablespoon Almond slivers
1 tablespoon grated fresh Ginger Root

Soak Shiitake Mushrooms in water for several hours. Strain, remove stems and cut up. Saute Mushrooms and Onions in Sesame Oil.
Add String Beans, Tarragon, Almond slivers and Ginger Root and a little water. Cover and simmer for 30 minutes.
Variations:
Use 1 teaspoon Savory and 1 T Turmeric instead of Tarragon.

GRAPE LEAVES FOR THE TABLE AND LUNCHBOX
(If you or your neighbor have a Grape Vine -- or you can buy them bottled in Middle Eastern markets.)

2 large chopped Onions
1 clove minced Garlic
4 tablespoon Olive Oil
1/4 cup fresh chopped Parsley
4 teaspoons chopped Dill Weed
1/4 cup Pine Nuts or slivered Almonds
2 tablespoon water
1 tablespoon Lemon Juice
2 cups cooked Rice

Saute Onions and Garlic in Olive Oil. Add Parsley, Dill, Nuts (Do not overheat oil.) Stir in water, Lemon Juice and cooked Rice. Mix and roll into Grape Leaves.
Variations:
Add 1/2 cup Raisins, 3/4 teaspoon Allspice, 1/2 teaspoon Cinnamon.

A "VITAMIN A" PLEASURE

Equal parts
Shredded orange/yellow
  Squash and 1 handful
  Carrots
Pumpkin or Squash Seeds

Mix Squash and Carrots. Toss in a handful of Seeds. Cover and steam 10 -15 minutes.
Variations:
Add other herbs according to need.
Whole Squashes (including the Seeds) can be slowly baked like a potato in the oven or they can be cut open and stuffed like a turkey before baking. (Hint: Speed up the baking process by first cutting the Squash in half and steaming the halves until slightly tender. Stuff with an herb-filled dressing and bake.)

A LIGHTER AND COOLING "SPAGHETTI"

2 cups fresh Bean Sprouts

Place Bean Sprouts in a strainer. Submerge for 15-30 seconds in a large pot of boiling water. Strain and use in place of spaghetti. Serve with a delicious sauce.
Variations:
Cut up and saute Bean Sprouts with Onion and liquid aminos in 2 tablespoon Sesame or Olive Oil. This can be mixed with other Herb/Vegetable dishes and/or eaten over a Grain.

INSTEAD OF POTATOES USE CASSAVA (YUCA)

Yuca Root
Water

Peel and rinse Yuca. Cut into quarters lengthwise and remove the fibrous cord. Place in a large enough pot to cover Yuca with Boiling Water. Simmer for 20-30 minutes or until tender. Remove from water and drain. Eat plain like a boiled Potato.
Variations:
Use in soups and stews. Mash like Potatoes.
Cover or mix with various sauces. Mix with Onions, Garlic and other herbs and form into patties for baking or pan browning.
Use Taro instead of Yuca or cook Yuca and Taro together.

INTERNAL SPRING CLEANING WITH BURDOCK ROOT

2 T Olive Oil
1 cup each scraped and
*   diagonally cut:*
*   Burdock Root*
*   Daikon Radish*
*   Parsnip*
*   Carrot*
2 cups shredded Cabbage
1/2 cup chopped Watercress
1 teaspoon Apple Cider
*   Vinegar*
1/4 cup water
1 T honey

Heat the Olive Oil and saute the Burdock Roots, Daikons, Parsnips and Carrots. Add Cabbage and Watercress. Mix the Cider Vinegar, Honey and Water together. Add to Vegetable saute. Stir and steam 10 minutes.

CACTUS TO STIMULATE INSULIN PRODUCTION

2 or 3 young, fresh Cactus
*   Pads*
1 large chopped Onion
1/2 cup diced Tomatoes
1/2 cup Corn
2 T Chili powder
1 teaspoon Apple Cider
*   Vinegar*
1/4 cup water

Peel and dice fresh Cactus Pads. Set aside. (Can use bottled precut Cactus.) Saute Onion. Add diced Cactus and vinegar. Cook till tender. Stir in Tomatoes, Corn, Chili powder and water. Cover and simmer for 15 minutes.
Serve over Rice.

A NUTRITIOUS VEGETABLE SANDWICH FOR THE LUNCHBOX

2 cups mixed chopped
*   Sprouts (include*
*   Sunflower seeds)*
1 cup cooked Rice
1/2 cup sliced Olives
1 cup Avocado

Mix ingredients with dressing of choice. Use as a stuffing to roll into a sheet or Nori Seaweed. (Hint: The rolled sheet will remain fastened by sealing the ends with a little water.) Wrap in waxed paper.
Variations:
Add chopped Nuts and/or Vegetables.
Use 2 slices of bread or a tortilla instead of Nori Seaweed.

THE SCOOP ON SOUPS

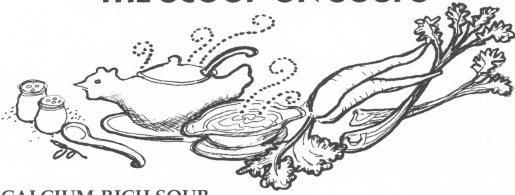

CALCIUM-RICH SOUP

2 cups Barley (soaked
   overnight and precooked)
1 chopped Onion
1 cup chopped Celery
1 cup chopped Kale
1 cup Sesame Nut Milk
   (see Beverages)

Combine ingredients. Cook 1 hour.
Blenderize for a creamy soup.

BLACK BEAN SOUP TO NOURISH LIVER AND BLOOD

2 cups dry Black Beans
2 cups chopped Onions
2 cloves Garlic
2 cups chopped Celery
1 cup shredded Carrots
1 cup cooked Rice
1/2 cup chopped Parsley
1/2 cup chopped
   Watercress
1/4 cup Black Sesame
   Seeds
Liquid aminos to taste

Soak 2 cups dry Black Beans 2 days. (Rinse
them thoroughly each day.) This causes
them to sprout, changing some of their
starch content to an easier to digest protein.
Add all other ingredients.
Cook in a crockpot or at low heat for 24-48
hours. Mash (or blend) part of the beans to
make a thicker, smoother soup.
Variations:
Add Spices according to taste and need.
   Some possibilities are Turmeric, Chili
   Powders, Cumin, Bay, Savory, Watercress,
   Parsley, fresh or canned Tomatoes.
After cooking and blending, add a textured
   Soy and/or Lentil Sprouts for a crunchier
   soup. Cook 1 hour longer.
Add 1/4 cup Peanut Butter.

POTASSIUM BROTH FOR FASTING

1 cup Zucchini
1 cup Potato Peels
1 cup chopped Watercress
1 tablespoon Seaweed
   Flakes
1 cup Carrot Peels

Slowly simmer ingredients in 2 quarts distilled water for 30-60 minutes. Or, cook overnight in a Crockpot on the lowest heat. Strain and drink the broth if on a fast. Or blenderize into a "cream" soup.

MISO TO ENHANCE DIGESTION AND BUILD BLOOD

1 tablespoon grated
   Ginger Root
4 chopped Green Onions
1/4 cup Seaweed flakes
2 tablespoon Miso paste

To 1 quart water add Onions, Ginger Root and Seaweed. Cook 30 minutes. Use 1/2 cup of soup mixture and Miso paste to make a gravy-like liquid. Add this thinned paste to the hot soup. Do not cook further.
Variations:
Add shredded Carrots, Zucchini or other
   Vegetables according to taste and need.
   Use this broth also to make sauces and
   cook Grains.

VEGETABLE SOUP FOR NUTRIENTS

1 cup chopped Celery
1 cup chopped Onions
1 cup sliced Carrots
1/2 cup each chopped:
   Bell Pepper
   Turnip Root
   Parsnips
   Cabbage
   Parsley
   Watercress
   Cilantro

Put ingredients in a large pot with 3 quarts of water. Add other herbs according to need and taste (Suggestions: Thyme, Basil, Savory, Sage, Cumin, Bay, Dil or Seaweed). Cover and slowly cook till done (about 2 hours).
Variations:
Add Okra, Tomatoes, Corn, Pea Pods,
   Bamboo Shoots, Greens and Yuca.

MOTHER'S MEDICINE FOR A (Cold Weather) COLD

1/4 cup coarsely chopped
   fresh Ginger Root
4 chopped Green Onions
2 cloves Garlic
2 cups diced Carrots
1/2 cup cooked Rice
1 tablespoon Thyme
1 teaspoon Sage
4 sprigs fresh or 2 T dry
   Lemongrass

Combine ingredients in 1/2 gallon water. Cook slowly till done. (Do not add cooling herbs to this soup.)
Variation:
Cut up 2 pieces untreated chicken – without skin.

PUMPKIN and MILLET SOUP TO RESTORE VIGOR

1 large can unsweetened
   Pumpkin
1/2 medium chopped
   Onion
1 pinch Clove powder
1/2 teaspoon Coriander
   powder
1 pinch of Nutmeg
1/2 teaspoon Cumin
1/4 cup Pumpkin Seeds
1/2 cup cooked Millet

Mix Pumpkin puree with enough water to thin it. Pour 1 1/2 cups of the liquid into a blender with Onion, Clove, Coriander, Cumin, Pumpkin Seeds and Millet. Blenderize all ingredients in this manner. Simmer 15 minutes. Serve with a dash of Nutmeg.
Variations:
Instead of canned Pumpkin, use 2 cups fresh cooked and mashed Pumpkin.

HEALTHFUL SPREADS

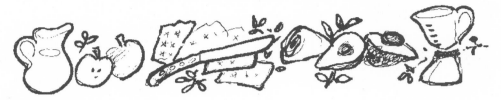

HUMMUS

1 cup cooked Garbanzo Beans
1 cup (2 day) sprouted
    (raw) Garbanzo Beans
1/4 cup Sesame Tahini
2 cloves pressed Garlic
2 tablespoon fresh Lemon
    Juice
2 tablespoon liquid aminos
1 1/2 cup water

Blenderize ingredients till smooth and creamy.
Variations:
Add mashed Avocado and 2 tablespoon white wine.
Use Miso soup instead of water.

NUTRITIOUS, PERFECT PROTEIN FOR THE LUNCHBOX

1 large Avocado
1 tablespoon Sesame Seed
meal
3 oz water or Juice

Blenderize ingredients for 30 seconds.
Variations:
Add Garlic, Chili Powder, Lemon Juice
    and/or honey.
Use as sandwich spread with Sprouts.
Add 1/4 cup 2 day old Sunflower Seed and
    Lentil Sprouts.

RESTORE YOUTH AND VITALITY WITH SEED SPREADS

1/4 cup each 2 day Sprouts:
    Sesame Seeds
    Sunflower Seeds
    Adzuki Beans
    Garbanzo Beans
    Lentils
1/4 cup Almonds soaked
    12 hours
2 Green Onions
1 clove Garlic
1/2 cup Tofu (Bean Curd)

1 tablespoon fresh Lemon
    Juice
2 T liquid aminos

Chop ingredients . Mix with Tofu, Lemon Juice and liquid aminos.
Variations:
Add other Herbs of your choice.
Add a mashed Avocado.
Use 1/4 cup Rejuvelac (see Beverages)
    instead of Tofu.

WARM THE MIDDLE WITH SPICY TUNA

1/2 cup baked, broiled or
  canned tuna
1/2 cup chopped Celery
1/2 cup chopped Bean
  Sprouts
2 chopped Green Onions
1 tablespoon Mustard
  (containing whole
  seeds)
2 tablespoon Curry
  Powder
2 tablespoon lowfat plain
  yogurt
2 tablespoon lowfat salad
  dressing

Thoroughly mix ingredients.
Variations:
Add 3 tablespoon Salsa.
Use albacore instead of tuna.
Add 1/2 cup String Beans.

APPLE-GINGER CHUTNEY

2 1/2 pounds large, cored,
  chopped Apples
1/2 cup chopped Ginger
  Root
1 1/2 cup honey
2 cups Apple Cider
  Vinegar
1/2 teaspoon each dry
  ground Cloves and
  Allspice
2 teaspoons ground
  Ginger
1/2 large finely chopped
  Onion
1/2 Lemon - peel grated,
  juice strained
1 cup Currants or Raisins

Place Vinegar, honey and spicy herbs into a large pot. Bring to a boil. Add Onions and Currants and cook 30 minutes. Add other ingredients and cook for an additional 30 minutes stirring frequently. Put into sterile canning jars. Cover and place jars into a large pot half filled with water. Put a lid on the pot and boil for 30 minutes. This and other Chutneys are a wonderful relish that aid digestion. (Makes about 4 pints and keeps for one year.)
Variations:
Add 1 cup Walnut pieces.

SALAD DRESSINGS WITH MEANING

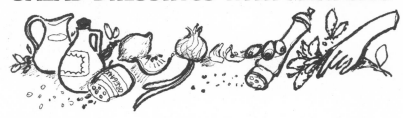

VINEGAR BASE - For making Dressings

Either Apple Cider, Rice or Malt Vinegar
A fresh Herb

Insert a large sprig of a fresh Herb into the bottle of Vinegar. (Select this Herb according to your needs and taste.) Close the bottle tightly and shake daily for 14 days. It will then be ready to use as a base for making your own dressing.

LEMON and OLIVE DRESSING – To stimulate liver functions

3 parts fresh Lemon Juice
1 part Olive Oil
1/2 part Flax Seed Oil
1/2 part water
1/4 cup dehydrated chopped Onion
1 clove pressed Garlic

Select other herbs according to need and taste. Cap and shake. Refrigerate.

LEMON - PARSLEY ITALIAN – To stimulate kidney functions

2 tablespoon each Olive Oil and Sesame Seeds
1 clove Garlic
2 tablespoon liquid aminos
2 teaspoons Apple Cider Vinegar
Juice of 2 Lemons
1/2 cup chopped fresh Parsley
1/4 teaspoon each dry Marjoram, Oregano and Savory

Blenderize first 6 ingredients. Then add herbs. Add water for a thinner dressing.

TAHINI DRESSING - A Tonic

1/2 cup Sesame Tahini
3 cloves Garlic
1/2 cup Lemon Juice
1/2 cup water
1/2 teaspoon liquid
    aminos
1/4 cup chopped fresh
    Parsley

Blenderize ingredients.
Variation:
Add other Herbs according to need and
    taste.

TOFU/AVOCADO DRESSING

1 large Avocado
1/4 cup Tofu
1/2 medium Onion
1 clove pressed Garlic
2 tablespoon Lemon Juice
1 tablespoon Worstershire
    Sauce
2 tablespoon liquid aminos

1 teaspoon each Savory
    and Parsley

Blenderize ingredients.

POPPY SEED DRESSING - For a relaxing evening meal

3 tablespoon white wine
Vinegar
1 tablespoon honey
1 tablespoon Mustard
2 tablespoon finely
minced Onion

1/4 cup Olive Oil
1 tablespoon Poppy Seeds
1 tablespoon Celery Seeds

Blenderize ingredients.

DRESSING - To aid the Colon

1 cup Sesame Tahini
1/4 cup Lemon Juice
1/4 cup Shredded raw Beet
1 clove minced Garlic
1 tablespoon Flax Seed
1 tablespoon chopped
Basil
2 tablespoon minced
Onion
1/4 cup liquid aminos

Blenderize ingredients till smooth.

SOULFUL SAUCES

ANTI-CANCER MUSHROOM SAUCE

1 cup (1/2 cup dried)
Shiitake Mushrooms
1 medium chopped Onion
2 tablespoon grated fresh
   Ginger Root
1 tablespoon Basil
2 tablespoon liquid
   aminos
2 tablespoon Taro flour or
   Cornstarch

Use fresh chopped or dried Shiitake Mushrooms. (Soak dried Mushrooms 1 hour in 2 cups water then finely chop.) Saute Onion and Ginger Root. Add Basil, liquid aminos, Shiitake Mushrooms along with the soak water. Simmer 15 minutes. Thicken by making a paste with Taro flour (available at most healthfood stores) or Cornstarch. Serve over Grains or Vegetables.

COOLING SALSA

1 cup Tomatoes
Chopped:
   1/2 cup Green Onions
   1/8 cup Green Peppers
   1/8 cup Cilantro
2 tablespoon Lemon Juice
1 teaspoon Chili Powder

Chop and mix ingredients.
Variations:
Add 2 tablespoon chunky Peanut Butter.
   Simmer 15 minutes.
Stir 1 tub Tofu, 2 tablespoon Mustard and
   1/4 teaspoon Turmeric into 1/2 the
   recipe. Use also as a sandwich Spread.

A SAUCE TO SPICE BLAND VEGETABLES

1/2 cup Lemon Juice
3 cloves finely minced
   Garlic
1 inch piece of grated
   Ginger Root
2 teaspoon pan toasted
   and ground Cumin
   Seeds
1/2 cup each, chopped
   Parsley and Cilantro

Thoroughly mix ingredients. Heat and use over steamed Vegetables.
Variations:
Add 1 tablespoon Mustard.
Use other Herbs according to need and
   taste.

AN HERBAL MARINADE FOR VEGETABLES, MEATS and/or GRAINS

*1 large can peeled, chopped
    Tomatoes*
1/8 cup Olive Oil
1/8 cup Flax Seed Oil
1 teaspoon Oregano
*1/4 teaspoon each Sage and
    Savory*
1/8 teaspoon Red Pepper
1/4 cup halved black olives
2 tablespoon capers

Mix ingredients and set aside 24 hours before using.

CURRY SAUCE FOR BETTER DIGESTION

4 tablespoon Sesame Oil
1 chopped Green Pepper
2 small chopped Onions
2 chopped Celery Stalks
1/2 cup chopped Mushrooms
1 small diced Zucchini
1 diced Carrot
2 tablespoon Curry Powder
3 cups Vegetable Stock
2 tablespoon Lemon Juice
1 tablespoon honey
*5 tablespoon Cornstarch or
Arrowroot*

Saute cut up Vegetables in Sesame Oil. Stir in Curry Powder and add Vegetable stock. Blenderize this mixture to a coarse texture, cover and simmer for 1 hour. Add Lemon Juice and honey. Then, thicken with Cornstarch or Arrowroot. (Make a paste with 1 cup of the Curry blend.) Bring to a boil. Reduce heat and simmer 15 minutes. Serve over Grains with Chutneys or fresh, chopped Papaya, Pineapple and Mango.
Variations:
Add 1 1/2 cups Grapes, 2 sliced Bananas. Serve over rice with chopped Almonds or Walnuts.

TOFU SAUCE

1/4 cup Sesame Seeds
1/2 cup water
1/4 cup liquid aminos
1/8 cup brewer's yeast flakes
*1/4 tablespoon each Kelp
    and Vegetable powders*
1/4 tablespoon Basil
1/2 clove mashed Garlic
*1 1/2 tablespoon Lemon
    Juice*
1 16 oz package rinsed Tofu

Blenderize ingredients until smooth and creamy. Use over steamed Vegetables or baked Tofu.
Variations:
Substitute Dulse Flakes for Kelp.
Use Almonds instead of Sesame Seeds.

LEAN ON BEANS

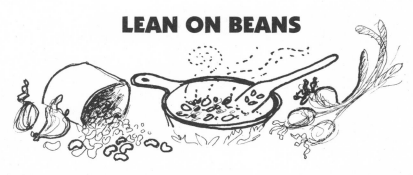

BEAN LOAF - A NUTRITIOUS MEAT SUBSTITUTE

2 cups cooked Beans
1 well beaten egg
1/2 cup Wholegrain
   Breadcrumbs
1/2 cup crumbled
   Wholegrain Cornbread
1 medium finely minced
   Onion
1 cup finely chopped
   Celery
1/4 cup finely chopped
   Green Pepper
2 tablespoon Sesame
   Seeds
1/2 cup cooked Quinoa
1 cup Miso Soup

Mix ingredients together. Shape into loaf and bake at 350 degrees for 30 minutes.

ADZUKI BEANS FOR STRONGER KIDNEYS

1 pound Adzuki Beans
3 quarts water
1 large Onion
1 clove pressed Garlic
1/2 teaspoon each Basil,
  Parsley, Savory, Marjoram
1/4 teaspoon grated Lemon
  Rind
1/8 cup liquid aminos
3 tablespoon Vegetable
  seasoning

Soak Adzuki Beans overnight, then drain. Adzuki Beans take longer to cook than other beans so begin by cooking them one hour before adding all other ingredients. Cook 2 additional hours or until beans are tender.
Variations:
Add 1/4 cup Black Sesame Seeds for
  greater kidney benefit.
After beans become tender, cook with equal
  part cooked Rice.

BACK TO BASIC BEANS
(FOR 1 POUND OF BEANS, LENTILS OR DRIED PEAS)

4 large chopped Onions
3 cloves pressed Garlic
1 large Green Pepper
(including seeds)
1 cup chopped Celery
1/2 cup each chopped
Celery Leaves and
Parsley
1 tablespoon each Mustard
Seeds and Chili powder
1 teaspoon Cumin
3 Bay Leaves
2 quarts of a nutritional
Herb tea made with
Alfalfa
1 tablespoon Apple Cider
Vinegar (to prevent gas)
1/4 cup liquid aminos

Combine all ingredients and cook several hours or till done. (Or cook 24 hours on "Low" in a Crockpot). All Beans should be soaked from 6 to 48 hours before cooking. To help prevent gas, freeze the soaked Beans before cooking. (When soaking over 6 hours, strain and rinse every few hours.)

Variations:

Add 1 large can Tomatoes, 1 small can Tomato Paste, 1/4 teaspoon ground Cinnamon, 2 whole Cloves, 1 cup grated Carrots.

If Mung Beans are used, add 4 T Curry Powder.

Use other Herbs according to need and taste.

MORE NUTRITIOUS SALADS

INSTEAD OF LETTUCE AND TOMATOES

A handful of each
chopped:
  Watercress
  Parsley
  Cilantro
  Alfalfa Sprouts
  Bean Sprouts
2 chopped Green Onions
1/4 small head shredded
  Cabbage
5 chopped spinach leaves

Mix ingredients well.
Variations:
Add 1 can tuna, 1/2 cup Olive halves,
  1 Avocado and 1 cup cooked Rice.

A SALAD TO SWEEP OUT THE INTESTINES

2 cups shredded Cabbage
1 cup shredded Carrots
1 cup grated Broccoli
  Stems
1/2 cup grated raw Beets
1/2 cup Fenugreek Sprouts

Mix ingredients well with an Olive Oil and
Lemon dressing.

PASTA/FENNEL WARMING SALAD

3 cups cooked Wholewheat
  and Vegetable pasta
1/2 cup each chopped
  Fennel Bulbs, Celery Root
5 finely chopped Green
  Onions
1/2 teaspoon each Sage and
  Thyme powders
1/4 cup chopped Fennel
  leaves

Toss all ingredients together and top with a
"lite" salad dressing; 2 T Mustard and 1 T
honey.

A SALAD TO EXTEND YOUTH AND VITALITY

On a bed of Alfalfa and/or Clover Sprouts arrange several kinds of 3 day Sprouts such as
- *Fenugreek*
- *Radish*
- *Garbanzo Beans*
- *Sunflower*
- *Lentils*
- *Cabbage*

HOW TO SPROUT: Put 4 T seeds in a large, wide-mouth jar. Cover the jar with cheese cloth and secure with a rubber band. Fill the jar with water and place in a dark place overnight. Pour water off. (Use this nutritious water on houseplants.) Rinse and drain the Sprouts 2 times daily for 2 to 4 days. After 4 days, refrigerate the Sprouts so they will not continue to grow and become tough.

MEAL-IN-ONE KIDNEY REJUVENATING SALAD

2 cups cooked Rice
1/2 cup each chopped Cauliflower and Dates
1 cup each chopped Celery and Apples
1/4 cup Sunflower Seed Sprouts
1/2 cup chopped Walnuts
1/2 cup chopped Parsley

Mix ingredients thoroughly and moisten with your desired amount of mayonnaise
Variations:
Use cooked Millet, cracked Wheat or mixed Grains instead of Rice.

TABOULI SALAD

2 cups cooked cracked Bulghur
1 cup chopped fresh Parsley
1 cup diced peeled Cucumber
1 cup finely minced Onion

Mix ingredients. Moisten with 1/4 cup Olive Oil mixed with 2 T Lemon Juice
Variations:
Add chopped Tomato to taste.
Use cooked Cous-Cous instead of Bulghur.

SIMPLE SWEET TREATS

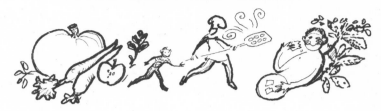

BLACK SESAME CANDY TO BUILD THE KIDNEYS

1 cup Black Sesame Seeds
2 tablespoon Lemon Juice
3/4 cup maple syrup

Heat syrup. Stir in Black Sesame Seeds and Lemon Juice. Press the mixture firmly into a moistened glassware cooking dish. Cool and cut into squares.
Variation:
Use molasses and honey instead of maple syrup.

USES FOR APPLE CONCENTRATE

2 tablespoon unflavored gelatin
1/2 cup boiling water
1/8 cup Apple concentrate
1 cup water

Dissolve gelatin in boiling water. Add Apple concentrate and 1 cup water. Chill.
Variations:
Add sliced Bananas and/or chopped Apples and Sunflower Seeds.
Add 1/4 cup Black Cherry concentrate.
Use 6 tablespoon Agar instead of gelatin. (Chilling is not necessary when using Agar.)
Use chopped Celery, shredded Carrots and other Vegetables instead of Fruits.
Instead of plain water, use an Herb tea made of Herbs according to need and taste.

BAKED APPLE

Sweet Apples
Raisins
Cinnamon and Nutmeg

Core large, naturally sweet Apples. Fill the cored centers with tightly packed raisins. Sprinkle with lots of Cinnamon and a dash of Nutmeg. Put in a covered baking dish. Bake at 350 degrees till tender.
Variations:
For a sweeter taste add 1 tablespoon maple syrup to each Apple.

UNSWEETENED APPLE SAUCE

1 quart cored, cut up
  Apples
1 cup water
3/4 cup Raisins
1/2 cup fresh squeezed
  Orange Juice
2 teaspoons Cinnamon
  powder

Steam Apples in a covered pan with 1 cup water till tender. Pulverize with a potato masher and add Raisins and Orange Juice. Cover and simmer 20 minutes.
Stir in Cinnamon.
Variations:
Add 3/4 cup chopped Walnuts or Sunflower Seeds.
To uncooked Apples add 1 cup chopped dry Apricots and/or Prunes and 1/2 cup additional water.

PUMPKIN PIE WITHOUT CRUST

1 large can (or 2 cups fresh)
  Pumpkin
1 pint of Carrot Juice
1 cup low-fat milk (optional)
1/2 cup pulverized raw
  Carrots
4 eggs slightly beaten
1/4 cup honey or maple
  syrup
2 teaspoons Ginger powder
1 tablespoon Cinnamon
  powder
1/2 teaspoon Allspice
1/4 teaspoon Clove powder

Blend ingredients thoroughly. Pour into shallow baking dishes and bake at 350 degrees for 1 hour or until done.
Variations:
Sprinkle with Sesame Seeds before baking.
Sprinkle with Granola after baking.
Use other Yellow and Orange Squashes.
Use Rice Dream or Koji (both commercial Rice products on sale at most healthfood stores) instead of milk.

FRUIT LEATHER

Papayas
Bananas
Pineapple

In a blender mix Papayas, Bananas and Pineapple. Pour onto a cookie sheet lined with waxed paper. Dry to a soft leathery texture using either a food dehydrator or an oven heated at 140 degrees. This process takes about 12 hours. Roll and cut into pieces.
Variations:
Use Melon mixes.
Use Berries mixed with Bananas.

GRAIN FLAN TO BUILD THE MIDDLE

6 tablespoon Agar Flakes
1 1/2 cups water
1 cup pureed and thinned (with water) Rice or Oatmeal porridge
3 tablespoon each maple syrup and honey
2 tablespoon Sesame tahini or Almond butter
2 teaspoons vanilla

Simmer Agar in water till dissolved. Blenderize with other ingredients and pour into individual dessert dishes.
Variations:
Serve with a "Caramel" sauce made of 4 tablespoon Barley malt, 2 teaspoons vanilla, 2 tablespoon water and 2 tablespoon maple syrup (Simmer till thickened and pour over each dish.).

DRY FRUIT CRUNCH BARS

2 cups finely chopped mixed dried Fruits
1 cup Cardamom tea
1/4 cup each coarsely chopped Sunflower Seeds, Sesame Seeds, Pumpkin Seeds, Walnuts, Almonds and Pine Nuts

Steam and mash dried Fruit (can use a combination of any type of dried Fruit). Mix with Seeds and Nuts. Press into an oiled glass dish. Cut into bars.
Variations:
Cover bars with unsweetened shredded Coconut or Sesame Seeds.

CAROB SYRUP TO REPLACE CHOCOLATE TOPPING

1/2 cup Carob powder
1/2 cup honey
3 tablespoon Almond or Walnut Oil
1 tablespoon Arrowroot powder (mixed with 1 tablespoon water)
1/2 cup boiling water
1 teaspoon vanilla
1 teaspoon Lemon Juice

Put Carob and Oil in pan. Add boiling water and mix. Stir in honey and Arrowroot mixture. Simmer 8 minutes. Cool. Add vanilla and Lemon Juice.

THE SAFE USE OF HERBS

YOUR RECIPES

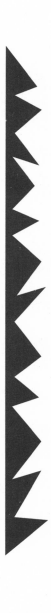

YOUR RECIPES

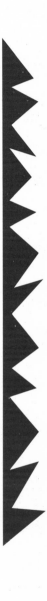

YOUR RECIPES

YOUR RECIPES

For Future Publications
Please send your favorite recipe creations to
NACHES PUBLICATIONS
590 Harmony Drive
Sedona, Arizona 86336

ELEVEN

APPENDIX

APPENDIX A

PRACTITIONERS TO CALL - HOLISTICALLY SPEAKING

Below is a brief description of various kinds of health care practitioners. Those who are most often educated in the use of healing herbs are pointed out (☛):

WESTERN CONVENTIONAL MEDICAL PRACTITIONERS*

- Medical Doctors (M.D., D.O.) - general practice, specialists and surgery
- Physician Assistants (P.A.) - assist Medical Doctors
- Nurse Practitioners (R.N.P.) - assist Medical Doctors or work independently
- Physical Therapists (P.T.) - assist Medical Doctors or work independently
- Dietitians (R.D.) - Nutritionists specializing in meal planning for institutions and medical patients
- Podiatrists (D.P.M.) - foot specialists (can do minor foot surgery)
- Dentists (D.D.S.) - general dental care and oral surgery
- Pharmacists - laboratory-made medicines (Some older pharmacists are familiar with Western herbs.)
- Optometrists (O.D.) - vision and prescription lens specialists
- Mental/Emotional Health Specialists: - Personal and Relationship Counseling
   Psychiatrists (M.D.)
   Psychologists (Ph.D.)
   Licensed Clinical Social Workers, (L.C.S.W.)
   Marriage, Family, Child Counselors (M.F.C.C.)

*The above medical practitioners are generally licensed in the states where they practice. Most health insurances cover their services.

WESTERN ALTERNATIVE MEDICAL PRACTITIONERS

- Chiropractors (D.C.) - spine and joint manipulations
- ☞ Naturopathic Doctors (N.D.) - detoxification, hydrotherapy, manipulation, natural medicines
- ☞ Homeopathic Doctors - use of herbal and mineral tinctures
- Nutritionists (B.S., M.S.) - use of foods and supplements to enhance wellness
- Colon Therapists - use of colonic irrigations to cleanse the colon
- Massage Therapists (M.T.) - use of European and polarity balancing massages

Of the above practitioners only Chiropractors are licensed in all states. Naturopathic physicians are licensed in only a few states. Most heath insurance companies cover Chiropractic. There are formal colleges and/or training centers for all of the above. Nutritionists should be health science graduates with 4 to 6 years university study.

NON-WESTERN MEDICAL PRACTITIONERS

- ☞ Acupuncturists/Herbalists - use needles, massage, herbs, diet and exercise
- ☞ Ayurvedic Doctors - use herbs, diet, massage, yoga, breathing, homeopathy, fasts
- ☞ Native American "Shamans" - use herbs, fasts, sweat baths, dance, ritual
- ☞ African/Carribean Doctors - use herbs, sound, ritual, dance, psychic powers
- Prayer Healers - use spiritual philosophies, affirmations, meditation, laying on of hands

Of the above practitioners only Acupuncturists are licensed in most states. Some are also formally trained Herbalists. Some insurance companies cover acupuncture.

IMPORTANT NOTES

The term "Holistic" refers to a collection of health care practices that come from various cultures (including Western conventional medical practices). Check the reputation and background of licensed and unlicensed practitioners before putting your life in their hands.

APPENDIX B
FOR ADDITIONAL INFORMATION:
SUGGESTED READING AND RESOURCES

ABOUT PROMOTING WELLNESS

Afua, Queen, *"Heal Thyself,"* A & B Books, Brooklyn, New York, 1992.

Beinfield, Harriet and Korngold, Efrem, *"Between Heaven And Earth — A Guide To Chinese Medicine,"* Ballantine Books, New York, 1991.

Chopra, Deepak, *"Perfect Health - The Complete Mind/Body Guide,"* Harmony Books (Division of Crown Publishers), New York, 1991.

Hay, Louise, *"You Can Heal Your Life,"* Hay House, Inc., Carson, Calif., 1987.

"NATURAL HEALTH — A Guide To Wellbeing," Published Bi-Monthly by Natural Health Limited Partnership, 17 Station Street, Box 1200, Brookline Village, Massachusetts, 02147.

"Wellness Made Easy - 101 Tips For Better Health," from the University of California, Berkeley Wellness Letter, School of Public Health, University of California at Berkeley, 1990.

ABOUT HERBS

Africa, Liaila, *"African Holistic Health,"* Sea Island Information Group (Adesegun, Johnson & Koram Publishers), Beltsville, Maryland, 1989.

BIO-DYNAMIC FARMING AND GARDENING ASSOCIATION, P.O. Box 550, Kimberton, Pennsylvania 19442. (Information about growing and eating organic produce.)

Heinerman, John, *"Encyclopedia of Fruits, Vegetables and Herbs,"* Parker Publishing Co., West Nyack, New York, 1988.

Heyn, Birgit, *"Ayurveda,"* (The Indian Art of Natural Medicine and Life Extension), Healing Arts Press, Rochester, Vermont, 1990.

Hutchens, Alma, *"Indian Herbalogy of North America,"* Merco, 620 Wyandotte East, Windsor 14, Ontario, Canada, 1973.

Mowrey, Daniel, *"The Scientific Validation of Herbal Medicine, (How To Remedy and Prevent Disease With Herbs, Vitamins, Minerals and*

Other Nutrients)" Keats Publishing, Inc., Connecticut, 1986.

SAN FRANCISCO HERB COMPANY, 250 14th Street, San Francisco, California 90220. (Wholesale/Retail source of culinary herbs and spices.)

THE HERB RESEARCH FOUNDATION, 1007 Pearl Street, Suite 200, Boulder, Colorado 80302. (Write for brochure and information.)

Ullman, Dana, et al., *"Everybody's Guide To Homeopathic Medicines (Taking Care of Yourself And Your Family With Safe And Effective Remedies),"* Jeremy P. Tarcher, Inc., Los Angeles, California, 1984.

ABOUT FOOD PREPARATION

Balch, James and Phyllis, *"Prescription For Cooking,"* PAB Books Publishing, Inc., Greenfield, Indiana, 1987.

" 'New Start' Homestyle," (All Natural Vegetarian Cooking) Weimar Institute, P.O. Box 486, Weimar, California 95736.

Turner, Kristina, *"The Self-Healing Cookbook - A Macrobiotic Primer For Healing Body, Mind and Moods With Whole, Natural Foods,"* Earthtones Press, Grass Valley, California 95945.

ABOUT TOXINS IN FOODS

Steinman, David, *"Diet For A Poisoned Planet - How To Choose Safe Foods For You And Your Family,"* Ballantine Books, New York, 1990.

Mott, Lawrie and Snyder, Karen, *"Pesticide Alert - A Guide To Pesticides In Fruits And Vegetables,"* Sierra Club Books, San Francisco, Ca., 1987.

ABOUT ALTERNATIVE PRACTITIONERS

Bonk, Melinda, Editor, *"Alternative Medicine Yellow Pages - The Comprehensive Guide to the New World of Health,"* Future Medicine Publishing, Inc., Puyallup, Washington, 1994.

INSTITUTE FOR TRADITIONAL MEDICINE (ITM) Researches the use of Chinese herbs in the treatment of various disorders. Also refers Eastern Medical practitioner/scholars across the country. 2017 S.E., Hawthorne, Portland, Oregon 97214.

WORLD RESEARCH FOUNDATION for a fee, searches out and prints worldwide collection of articles on any disorder—including holistic practitioners. 15300 Ventura Blvd., Suite 405, Sherman Oaks 91403.

APPENDIX C
BOTANICAL NAMES

Agar Agar .... *Agar*
Alfalfa .... *Medicago sativa*
Allspice ...... *Pimenta officinalis*
Almond ...... *Prunus amygdalus*
Aloe .... *Aloe vera*
Amaranth .... *Amaranthus hypochondriacus*
Anise .... *Pimpinella Anisum*
Apple .... *Pyrus malus*
Apricot ..... *Prunus armeniaca*
Arrowroot .... *Maranta arundinacea*
Artichoke .... *Cynara scolymus*
Asparagus ... *Asparagus officinalis*
Avocado ..... *Persea americana*
Bamboo
Shoots .... *Bambusa beecheyana*
Banana ...... *Musa sapien*
Barley .... *Hordeum vulgare*
Basil .... *Ocimum basilicum*
Bay .... *Laurus nobilis*
Beans .... *Phaseolus genus*
Beet Root ..... *Beta vulgaris*
Broccoli ..... *Brassica oleracea italica*
Buckwheat ... *Fagopyrum vulgare*
Burdock Root . *Arctium lappa*
Cabbage ..... *Brassica oleracea*
Caraway ..... *Carum carvi*
Cardamom ... *Elettaria cardamomum*
Carob .... *Ceratonial siliqua*
Carrot .... *Daucus carota*
Cassava (Yuca) *(several varieties) Manihot esculenta*
Cauliflower ... *Brassica oleracea botrytis*

Cayenne ..... *Capsicum frutescens*
Celery .... *Apium graveolens*
Chamomile ... *Anthemis nobilis*
Cherry .... *Prunus avium*
Chestnut ..... *Heleocharis tuberosa*
Chives .... *Allium schoenoprasum*
Cinnamon .... *Cinnamomum cassia*
Cloves .... *Eugenia caryophyllata Syzygium aromaticum*
Coconut ...... *Cocos nucifera*
Collards ...... *Brassica oleracea acephala*
Coriander .... *Coriandrum sativum*
Corn .... *Zea Mays*
Cornsilk ..... *Zea Mays*
Cranberry .... *Vaccinium macrocarpum*
Cucumber .... *Cucumis sativus*
Cumin .... *Cuminum cyminum*
Currants ..... *Ribes nigrum*
Dandelion .... *Taraxicum officinale*
Dill .... *Anethum graveolens*
Dulse .... *Rhodymenia palmata*
Fennel .... *Foeniculum vulgare*
Fig .... *Ficus carica*
Flax Seeds .... *Linus usitatissimum*
Foenugreek ... *Trigonella foenum-graecyn*
Garlic .... *Allium sativum*
Ginger .... *Zingiber officinale*
Grapefruit .... *Citrus paradisi*
Grapes .... *Vitis species*
Hazelnuts .... *Corylus avellana pontica*

Horseradish	*Armoracia lapathifolia*	Rye	*Secale cereale*
Kale	*Brassica oleracea acephala*	Safflower	*Carthamus*
		Saffron	*Crocus sativus*
Kelp	*Fucus vesiculosus*	Sage	*Salvia officinalis*
Leek	*Allium porrum*	Savory	*Satureja*
Lemon	*Citrus limon*	Sesame	*Sesamum indicum*
Lemongrass	*Cymbopogon citratus*	Shiitake	*Lentinus edodes*
Mango	*Mangifera indica*	Soya	*Soja max*
Marjoram	*Majorana hortenses*	Sunflower	*Helianthus annuus*
Millet	*Panicum milliaceum*	Swiss Chard	*Beta Vulgaris cicla*
Mints	*Mentha*	Tangerines	*Citrus reticulata*
Mustard	*Brassica hirta*	Taro Root	*(several varieties)*
Nutmeg	*Myristica gragrans*	Tarragon	*Artemisia dracunculus*
Oat	*Avena sativa*	Thyme	*Thymus vulgaris*
Olive	*Olea europaea*	Tomato	*Lycopersicon esculentum*
Onion	*Allium cepa*		
Oranges	*Citrus sinensis*	Turmeric	*Curcuma longa*
Oregano	*Lippia*	Walnuts	*Juglans regia*
Papaya	*Carica papaya*	Watercress	*Nasturtium officinale*
Paprika	*Capsicum annuum*	Watermelon	*Citrullus vulgaris*
Parsley	*Petroselium crispum*	Wheat	*Triticum aestivum*
Peanut	*Archis hypogaea*	Yucca	*Yucca liliaceae and agavaceae*
Pear	*Pyrus Bretschneideri*		
Persimmons	*Diospyros dumetorum*		
Pinapple	*Ananas comosus*		
Pinenut	*Pinus koraienses*		
Pomegranate	*Punica granatum*		
Poppy Seeds	*Papaver somniferum*		
Potato (Sweet)	*Ipomea batatas*		
Potato (White)	*Solanum tuberosum*		
Pumpkin	*Cucurbita moschata*		
Quinoa	*Chenopodium quinoa*		
Radish	*Raphani sativus*		
Reishi	*Ganoderma lucidum*		
Rice	*Oryza sativa*		
Rosemary	*Rosmarinus officinalis*		

INDEX

BURNOUT 24

BREATHING EXERCISES 48-55

COLON IRRIGATION 54

COLON STIMULATOR 54 -55, 59, 69, 71, 72, 88

FASTING 38, 52, 106

FDA GUIDELINES 3, 5

HERBALISTS 2-3

HERBS (COMMON HOUSEHOLD)

Agar 10, 23, 25, 55, **59**

Alfalfa 10, 17, 23, 25, 39, 51, 53, 54, 55, **59**, 98

Allspice 10, 19, **59**

Aloe Vera 17, 47, 53, 55, **59-60**, 100

Amaranth **75**

Anise 10, 19, **60**

Arrowroot **91**

Artichokes 39, **91**

Asparagus 51, **92**

Avocados **70**

Bamboo Shoots 10, 21, **60**

Barley 17, 21, **75-76**

Basil 10, 25, 37, 47, 51, 53, 55, **61**, 98

Bay (Laurel) 10, 37, 47, 53, **61**, 98

Bean Sprouts (See Sprouts)

Beans (See Legumes) 10, 21, 55, **79-80**, 100

Beets 10, 52, 54, 55, **92**

Broccoli 37, 98

Buckwheat 10, 19, **76**

Burdock Root 10, 17, 39, 47, 53, 55, **62**, 99, 100

Cabbage 37, 54

Cactus Pads 10, 21, **62**

Caraway 10, 21, **62**

Cardamom 10 ,19, 21, 37, 51, **63**

Carob 21, **79**

Carrots 37, 52, **92**

Cassava (See Yucca) 93

Cauliflower 37, 98

Cayenne Pepper 10, 19, 37, 47, 49, **63**

Celery 10, 17, 23, 25, 39, 51, 52, **64**, 99, 100

Chamomile 39, 53, 54, **64-65**, 98

Cherries 25, **70**

Chia Seeds 86, 98

Chives 10, 37, 49, **65**

Cilandro (See Coriander)

Cinnamon 10, 19, 25, 31, 37, 47, 49, **65-66**, 87, 99

Citrus 52, **70-71**

Cloves 19, 25, 51, **66**, 69, 98

Coconut 23, 25, **70-71**

Coriander 25, 53, **66**, 98

Corn **76**

Cornsilk 17, 21, **66-67**

Cranberries 51, 67, **71**

Cucumbers **17**

Cumin 25, **67**

Dandelion (See Greens)

Dill 10, 25, 53, **67**

Dry Fruits 55, **71**

Fennel 10, 19, 21, 25, 37, 49, 51, 53, 55, **67-68**

Fenugreek Seed 10, 19, 21, 25, 37, 49, 51, 53, 55, **67-68**

Flax Seed 10, 51, 53, 54, 55, **69**, 88, 98

Fruits (Common Fresh) 25, 55, **69-70**, 99

Garlic 10, 37, 39, 47, 49, 55, **73-74**

Ginger 10, 19, 31, 37, 47, **74**

Grains 25, 51, 55, **75**

Grape Leaves 17

Grapefruit (See Citrus)

Grapes 39, **71-72**

Greens 17, 53, 55, **78**, 98, 100

Greens 25, 39, 54, **78**

Horseradish 10, 19, 49, **78**

Kale **92**

Legumes 54, 55, 10, 21, 55, **79**

Lemon 17, 39, 53, 70, **72**, 100

Lemongrass 25, 39, 53, **80**, 98

Loquats 23, **72**

Mace 83

Marjoram 10, 25, 31, 49, 51, **80-81**, 98

Melons 23, **72**

Millet 76

Mint 10, 17, 33, 37, 47, 49, **81**, 98

Mushrooms 81

Mustard Seeds 10, 19, 49, **82**

Nutmeg 10, 19, **82-83**

Nuts 23, 25, 51, 52, 55, **83**

Oats 51, **76**

Olive Oil 88

Onions 10, 19, 47, 49, **83-84**

Orange Peels 49, 84

Oregano 10, 25, 31, 49, 84

Paprika 64

Parsley 17, 21, 25, 39, 51, 53, 66, **84**, 98, 99

Parsnips 99

Peanuts **79**

Persimmons 23, **72**

Pineapple 37, **72-73**

Pomegranates 25, 51, **73**

Poppy Seeds 23, 55, 75, **85**

Potato 93, 99

Prickly Pears 21

Pumpkin Seeds 10, 75, **85**

Quinoa 51, **76**

Radishes 92

Rice 51, 21, **76**

Rosemary 10, 25, 39, 53, **85**, 98

Rye 51, 76

Safflower 37, **86**

Saffron 37, **86**, 88

Sage 10, 19, 25, 31, 39, 47, 51, **86**, 98

Savory 10, 19, 25, 39, 51, **86**

Seaweeds 10, 19, 39, **86**, 98, 100

Sesame Seeds 10, 23, 25, 55, 75, **86-87**, 98

Soya Beans **80**

Sprouts 17, 23, 54, 55, **61**, 98

Sunflower 10, 25, 75, **88-89**

Taro Root 10, 17, 21, **89**

Tarragon 10, 21, **89**

Thyme 10, 25, 31, 47, 49, **89-90**

Tomatoes **73**

Tropical Fruits **73**

Turmeric 10, 17, 37, 53, **90**

Turnips 99

Vegetables (Common Fresh) 25, 55, **91**

Watercress 17, 25, 39, 47, 49, 51, 53, **90**, 98

Watermelon 17, 21, 51, **90-91**
Wheat 51, **76**
Yucca (Yuca) 39, 51, **92-93**, 99
HERBS
    Classification of 15
    Nutritive Value of 4, 5
    Preparation of 96-136
    Selection of 15
    Unsafe Use of 2-5
    Where to Find 29, 144-145

IDEAL WELLNESS CHECKLIST xii-xiv

INTERNAL IMBALANCES
    Heat 16-17, 32-33
    Cold 18-19, 30-31
    Damp 20-21
    Dry 22-23
    Self-abuse 24-25
KITCHEN CONVENIENCES 104-105

NERVES (Relaxation of) 61, 64, 65, 76,
    80-81, 85, 86, 90

OFFICE OF ALTERNATIVE
    MEDICINE 3

ORGANS OF ELIMINATION
    Blood 40
    Bowel/Colon 54-55, 41
    Kidneys 50-51, 41
    Liver 38-39, 52-53, 41
    Lung 48-49, 41
    Lymphatic System 36
    Skin 46-47, 41

PARTS OF PLANTS 97

RECIPES FOR WELLNESS
Daily Basic Guideline: Meal
    Building 107
Beverages
    Seed Milk 110
    Make Your Own Sodas 110
    Smoothy 110
    Purposeful Beverages 111
    Warm the Middle Ginger Drink 111
    Rejuvelac Milk Substitute 111
    Digestion Warming Tea 112
    Nerve Tonic 112
    Cleansing/Fasting Juice 112

    In From the Cold Air 112
Grains
    Mixed Grain for Total Nutrition 113
    Rice Cereal for Nourishing Ill and
        Children 113
    Spiced Rice 113
    Vegeburger 114
    Granola for Digestion 114
    Nutloaf 114
    Cornbread Plus 115
    Pilaf for Health 114
    Kasha - Cold Weather Warmer 115
    Wild Rice for Nerves and
        Glands 116
    Millet for Digestion and Immune
        Functions 116
Vegetables
    Nourishing African Greens 117
    Alleged Cancer Fighter 117
    Cleanse the Bowel 118
    To Warm and Dry and Middle 118
    Grape Leaves 118
    Vitamin A Pleasure 119
    A Lighter/Cooling "Spaghetti" 119
    Instead of Potatoes Use Cassava 119
    Internal Cleaning with Burdock
        Root 120
    Cactus to Stimulate Insulin 120
    Nutritious Vegetable Sandwich 120
Soups
    Calcium Rich 121
    Black Bean to Nourish Liver
        and Blood 121
    Potassium Broth For Fasting 122
    Miso to Enhance Digestion and
        Build Blood 122
    Vegetable Soup For Nutrients 122
    Mother's Medicine For A Cold 123
    Pumpkin and Millet Soup To
        Restore Vigor 123
Spreads
    Hummus 124
    Nutritious Perfect Protein For the
        Lunchbox 124
    Restore Youth and Vitality With
        Seed Spreads 124
    Warm the Middle With Spicy
        Tuna 125

    Apple-Ginger Chutney 125
Salad Dressings
    Vinegar Base 126
    Lemon and Olive to Stimulate
        Liver 126
    Lemon and Parsley to Stimulate
        Kidneys 126
    Tahini - A Tonic 127
    Tofu/Avacado 127
    Poppy Seed For a Relaxing Meal 127
    Dressing to Aid the Colon 127
Sauces
    Anti-Cancer Mushroom 128
    Cooling Salsa 128
    To Spice Bland Vegetables 128
    Herbal Marinade For Vegetables/
        Meats/Grains 129
    Tofu 130
Beans
    Bean Loaf - A Nutritious Meat
    Substitute 130
    Adzuki Beans for Stronger
        Kidneys 130
    Back to Basic Beans 131
Salads
    Instead of Lettuce and
        Tomatoes 132
    To Sweep Out the Intestines 132
    Pasta/Fennel Warming Salad 132
    To Extend Youth and Vitality 133
    Meal-In-One Kidney
    Rejuvenating 133
    Tabouli 133
Sweets
    Black Sesame Candy to Build
        Kidneys 134
    Uses for Apple Concentrate 134
    Baked Apple 134
    Unsweetened Applesauce 135
    Pumpkin Pie Without Crust 135
    Fruit Leather 135
    Grain Flan To Build the Middle 136
    Dry Fruit Crunch Bars 136
    Carob Syrup to Replace Chocolate
        Topping 136

SPICES 4

WORLD HEALTH ORGANIZATION 58

ABOUT THE AUTHOR

BEVERLY E. COLEMAN received a B.A. in Sociology/Anthropology from Cal State University at Los Angeles in 1961 and a Master's Degree in Public Health from U.C.L.A. in 1969. In 1987 she was awarded a M.S. in Traditional Chinese Medicine from Emperor's College in Santa Monica, California where she later joined the staff as a Professor of Herbology. She is licensed by The State of California to practice Herbology and Acupuncture and is an Acupuncture Diplomat certified by the National Certification Board. The author has lived, and studied in Native American, African, Asian and European cultures. Many of the author's unique presentations of herbs and nutrition herein reflect both a scholarly and practical knowledge of multi-cultural approaches to health and herbal science. The author is presently an Acupuncturist/Herbalist in private practice in Los Angeles, California and Sedona, Arizona. she also writes, lectures and teaches in community settings and at local colleges on various health related topics and is the author of the *"Coleman Wellness Self Test."*

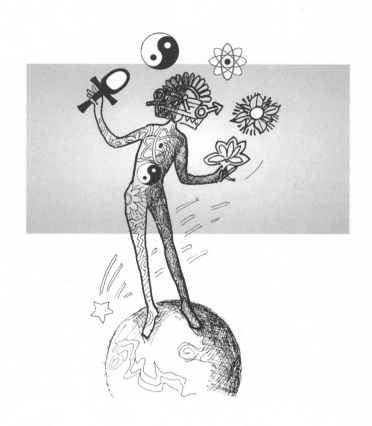

ORDER FORM

To order **THE SAFE USE OF HERBS** or receive information about other NACHES PUBLICATIONS, write:

NACHES PUBLICATIONS
590 Harmony Drive
Sedona, Arizona 86336
or Telephone:
Telephone (520) 204-9233
Fax (520) 204-2027
To order in the Los Angeles, California area call: (310) 558-0164

Ship To: (Name) _____

Address _____ Unit # _____

City _____ State _____ Zip _____

Phone _____

_____ No. of copies @ $15.95 per copy

Amount for Books . . . .   _____

Shipping/Handling

$2.50 first book . . . .   _____

50 cents ea. additional book . . . . . .   _____

State Tax (if applicable) . . . .   _____

TOTAL AMOUNT DUE   _____

Method of payment:
❑ Check
❑ Money Order
❑ Visa/Mastercard

Card # _____ Expiration _____

Name on Card (Print) _____

Signature: _____

*Retailers please call for wholesale ordering information